Rhinoplasty: Current Therapy

Guest Editors

Shahrokh C. Bagheri, DMD, MD, FACS
Husain Ali Khan, MD, DMD
Angelo Cuzalina, MD, DDS

ORAL AND MAXILLOFACIAL SURGERY CLINICS OF NORTH AMERICA

www.oralmaxsurgery.theclinics.com

Consulting Editor
RICHARD H. HAUG, DDS

February 2012 • Volume 24 • Number 1

SAUNDERS an imprint of ELSEVIER, Inc.

W.B. SAUNDERS COMPANY
A Division of Elsevier Inc.

1600 John F. Kennedy Blvd. • Suite 1800 • Philadelphia, PA 19103-2899

www.oralmaxsurgery.theclinics.com

ORAL AND MAXILLOFACIAL SURGERY CLINICS OF NORTH AMERICA Volume 24, Number 1
February 2012 ISSN 1042-3699, ISBN-13: 978-1-4557-3902-8

Editor: John Vassallo; j.vassallo@elsevier.com
Developmental Editor: Teia Stone

Oral and Maxillofacial Surgery Clinics of North America (ISSN 1042-3699) is published quarterly by Elsevier Inc., 360 Park Avenue South, New York, NY 10010-1710. Months of issue are February, May, August, and November. Business and Editorial Offices: 1600 John F. Kennedy Blvd., Suite 1800, Philadelphia, PA 19103-2899. Periodicals postage paid at New York, NY and additional mailing offices. Subscription prices are $355.00 per year for US individuals, $522.00 per year for US institutions, $159.00 per year for US students and residents, $414.00 per year for Canadian individuals, $621.00 per year for Canadian institutions, $476.00 per year for international individuals, $621.00 per year for international institutions and $216.00 per year for Canadian and foreign students/residents. To receive student/resident rate, orders must be accompanied by name or affiliated institution, date of term, and the *signature* of program/residency coordinator on institution letterhead. Orders will be billed at individual rate until proof of status is received. Foreign air speed delivery is included in all *Clinics* subscription prices. All prices are subject to change without notice. **POSTMASTER:** Send address changes to *Oral and Maxillofacial Surgery Clinics of North America,* Elsevier Periodicals Customer Service, 11830 Westline Industrial Drive, St. Louis, MO 63146. Tel: 1-800-654-2452 (U.S. and Canada); 314-447-8871 (outside U.S. and Canada). Fax: 314-447-8029. E-mail: journalscustomerservice-usa@elsevier.com (for print support); journalsonlinesupport-usa@elsevier.com (for online support).

Reprints. For copies of 100 or more, of articles in this publication, please contact the Commercial Reprints Department, Elsevier Inc., 360 Park Avenue South, New York, NY 10010-1710. Tel.: 212-633-3812; Fax: 212-462-1935; Email: reprints@elsevier.com.

Oral and Maxillofacial Surgery Clinics of North America is covered in MEDLINE/PubMed (*Index Medicus*).

Printed and bound by CPI Group (UK) Ltd, Croydon, CR0 4YY

Transferred to Digital Print 2012

Contributors

CONSULTING EDITOR

RICHARD H. HAUG, DDS
Carolinas Center for Oral Health,
Charlotte, North Carolina

GUEST EDITORS

SHAHROKH C. BAGHERI, DMD, MD, FACS
Chief, Division of Oral and Maxillofacial
Surgery, Department of Surgery, Northside
Hospital, Atlanta; Clinical Associate Professor,
Department of Oral and Maxillofacial Surgery,
Georgia Health Sciences University, Augusta;
Clinical Assistant Professor, Department of
Surgery, School of Medicine, Emory University,
Atlanta; Georgia Oral and Facial Surgery, and
Eastern Surgical Associates and Consultants,
Atlanta, Georgia

HUSAIN ALI KHAN, MD, DMD
Attending Surgeon, Division of Oral and
Maxillofacial Surgery, Department of Surgery,
Northside Hospital, Atlanta; Georgia Oral and
Facial Surgery, and Eastern Surgical
Associates and Consultants, Atlanta;
Aesthetics International USA, Atlanta; Clinical
Associate Professor, Department of Oral and
Maxillofacial Surgery, Georgia Health
Sciences, Augusta, Georgia

ANGELO CUZALINA, MD, DDS
Associate Faculty, Oklahoma State University
Center for Health Sciences; Private Practice,
Tulsa Surgical Arts, Tulsa, Oklahoma

AUTHORS

SHAHROKH C. BAGHERI, DMD, MD, FACS
Chief, Division of Oral and Maxillofacial
Surgery, Department of Surgery, Northside
Hospital, Atlanta; Clinical Associate Professor,
Department of Oral and Maxillofacial Surgery,
Georgia Health Sciences University, Augusta;
Clinical Assistant Professor, Department of
Surgery, School of Medicine, Emory University,
Atlanta; Georgia Oral and Facial Surgery, and
Eastern Surgical Associates and Consultants,
Atlanta, Georgia

MOHAMMAD BAYAT, DMD
Department of Oral and Maxillofacial Surgery,
Shariati Hospital, Tehran University of Medical
Sciences, Tehran, Iran

LOUIS S. BELINFANTE, DDS
Private Practice, Dawsonville, Georgia

BEHNAM BOHLULI, DMD
Department of Oral and Maxillofacial Surgery,
Buali Hospital, Azad University,
Tehran, Iran

ANGELO CUZALINA, MD, DDS
Associate Faculty, Oklahoma State University
Center for Health Sciences; Private Practice,
Tulsa Surgical Arts, Tulsa, Oklahoma

R. CHAD DEAL, MD
Southern Surgical Arts, Lookout Mountain,
Georgia

JAMES D'SILVA, MCH, DNB
Consultant, The Cosmetic Surgery Institute,
Bandra-West; Consultant, Cosmetic Surgery,
Breach Candy Hospital, Mumbai,
Maharashtra, India

HANY A. EMAM, BDS, MS
Chief Resident, Department of Oral and Maxillofacial Surgery, Georgia Health Sciences University, Augusta, Georgia

HUSAIN ALI KHAN, MD, DMD
Attending Surgeon, Division of Oral and Maxillofacial Surgery, Department of Surgery, Northside Hospital, Atlanta; Georgia Oral and Facial Surgery, and Eastern Surgical Associates and Consultants, Atlanta; Aesthetics International USA, Atlanta; Clinical Associate Professor, Department of Oral and Maxillofacial Surgery, Georgia Health Sciences, Augusta, Georgia

JAMES KOEHLER, MD, DDS
Adjunct Clinical Assistant Professor of Surgery, Oklahoma State University; Private Practice, Tulsa Surgical Arts, Tulsa, Oklahoma

LANDON MCLAIN, MD, DMD
Private Practice, Carolinas Center for Cosmetic Surgery, Charlotte, North Carolina

NIMA MOHARAMNEJAD, DMD
Craniomaxillofacial Research Center, Shariati Hospital, Tehran University of Medical Sciences, Tehran, Iran

L. MIKE NAYAK, MD
Nayak Plastic Surgery and Skin Enhancement Center; Clinical Assistant Professor, Department of Otolaryngology–Head and Neck Surgery, Saint Louis University, St Louis, Missouri

CAREY J. NEASE, MD
Southern Surgical Arts, Lookout Mountain, Georgia

JASON K. POTTER, MD, DDS
Private Practice, Plastic Surgery, Dallas, Texas

CLEMENT QAQISH, DDS, MD
Private Practice, North County Cosmetic Surgery, Escondido, California

MARY L. SCHINKEL, DO
PGY5 Otorhinolaryngology Resident, Department of Medical Education, Des Peres Hospital, St Louis, Missouri

MARK R. STEVENS, DDS
Professor and Chairman, Oral and Maxillofacial Surgery Department, Georgia Health Sciences University, Augusta, Georgia

MOHAN THOMAS, MD, DDS
Senior Consultant, The Cosmetic Surgery Institute, Bandra-West; Senior Consultant, Cosmetic Surgery, Breach Candy Hospital, Mumbai, Maharashtra, India

PETER D. WAITE, MPH, DDS, MD
Professor and Chairman, Department of Oral and Maxillofacial Surgery, University of Alabama at Birmingham, Birmingham, Alabama

AMIN YAMANI, DMD
Department of Oral and Maxillofacial Surgery, Buali Hospital, Azad University, Tehran, Iran

Contents

Man has considered the nose to be a key feature, if not the key feature, of facial appearance, beauty, and dynamics. However, because of its central facial location and weak cartilaginous support, the nose is susceptible to disfiguring infection, trauma, pathologic entities, and human-associated carnages. This article discusses the various methods (eg, endonasal approach, external approach, and osteoplastic operations) surgeons have tried throughout history to give their patients a more attractive face by altering the one physical anatomic structure that one usually notices first.

Many cosmetic surgeons consider rhinoplasty to be the most complex surgical and artistically challenging of all aesthetic surgery today. It is the most common facial procedure performed for women and the second most common for men. The art and science of cosmetic rhinoplasty begins with the initial examination. The surgeon must visualize and predict like Leonardo Da Vinci, be a sculptor like Michelangelo, and be an analyzer like Einstein. This article describes the components and complexities of the initial examination in cosmetic rhinoplasty.

Although anatomy often seems static, the continual innovation of new surgical techniques and approaches, in reality, make it a dynamic field. The first essential principal of any surgery is the comprehensive knowledge of the anatomic area and its physiology. This assertion is especially true in functional and or cosmetic nasal surgery.

The last 2 decades have witnessed significant changes in both technical and philosophic aspects of rhinoplasty surgery. Many of these changes are designed to provide more predictable, lasting, and enhanced cosmetic results of surgery without compromise of function. Although the aim of this procedure remains unchanged, the techniques and methodology have evolved. What is also continuously changing is the patients' requests and expectations of favorable cosmetic outcome. This article outlines the basic concepts that are essential in performing cosmetic rhinoplasty.

This article discusses the intimate relationship that the form of the nasal septum and the esthetics of the nose have with one another and that alterations of either can significantly affect the other. Surgeons from several specialties perform surgical alterations of the external and internal nose; however, many of the advancements have been kept within the literature of their respective fields. It would be wise for rhinoplasty surgeons to have solid understanding of the form and function of the nose so that they may bridge the gaps of their specialty and provide the best possible care for their patients.

As rhinoplasty techniques continue to evolve toward structural support and away from purely reductive techniques, the need for sophisticated grafting options will escalate to augment or replace critical support mechanisms of the nose. This will result in improved esthetic outcomes and functional results. We have found that well-planned and executed adjunctive grafting techniques can deliver lasting results with preservation of function and cosmesis. This article reviews the various graft materials and the techniques and indications for their use.

Rhinoplasty remains a challenging art but is now systematized at least in part by recent understanding of the supporting mechanisms and how they may be manipulated to control the nasal tip. Nasal tip control is the key to a successful, aesthetically pleasing, rhinoplasty result with preservation of nasal function.

Lateral osteotomy is a controversial step in rhinoplasty, which is usually performed to narrow a wide nose, widen a narrow bony pyramid, straighten a deviated nose, or close an open roof deformity. The osteotomy is performed using several methods, although the internal continuous and external perforator are the main ways to perform the lateral osteotomy. Most other techniques are modifications of these basic methods. The purpose of this article is to review the essential concepts of nasal hump surgery and lateral osteotomy as used in cosmetic rhinoplasty.

The nasal base is an important aspect of the nose with a complex anatomic architecture comprising a combination of cartilages, skin, connective tissues, and ligaments. Recent studies show that all nasal base deformities cannot be corrected by simple excision and suturing techniques. Alar release and medialization would be effective in some of these deformities. This article presents an overview of conventional concepts of alar base surgeries, which have remained unchanged over many years. Indications and limitations of each technique are discussed, followed by a more detailed description of alar release and medialization.

Correction of the deviated nose is one of the most difficult tasks in rhinoplasty surgery and should be approached in a systematic manner to ensure a satisfied patient and surgeon. Correction of the deviated nose is unique in that the patient's complaints frequently include aesthetic and functional characteristics. Equal importance should be given to the preoperative, intraoperative, and postoperative aspects of the patient's treatment to ensure a favorable outcome.

Oral and Maxillofacial Surgery Clinics of North America

RELATED INTEREST

Facial Plastic Surgery Clinics of North America, February 2011 (Vol. 19, No. 1)
Nasal Reconstruction
Daniel G. Becker, MD, *Guest Editor*

THE CLINICS ARE NOW AVAILABLE ONLINE!
Access your subscription at:
www.theclinics.com

Preface
Rhinoplasty: Current Therapy

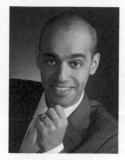

Shahrokh C. Bagheri,
DMD, MD

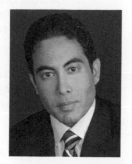

Husain Ali Khan, MD, DMD

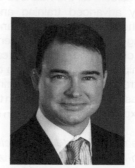

Angelo Cuzalina, MD, DDS

Guest Editors

Like any surgical procedure, rhinoplasty has evolved based on improved surgical techniques that survived the test of time and patients' increasing expectations. As in most cosmetic procedures, the vast majority of advances for rhinoplasty are from the teachings of surgical skill sets to younger surgeons through operative training, textbooks, lectures, and symposia. The difficulty of developing randomized or prospective cohort studies and multi-center analysis for cosmetic procedures contributes to the progression via traditional (non-research-based) modes of teaching. Cosmetic surgery is unique among other surgical specialties due to changing trends and racial and regional ethnic preferences that drive patients' desires to what is considered an esthetic result. In no other procedure are such differences as clear as for rhinoplasty. The operation is individually customized with respect to current ethnic and cultural norms. In modern rhinoplasty surgery, no single procedure or approach can provide a reproducible outcome for the vast array of patient desires for beauty and functionality. Surgeons have to be armed with multiple techniques that are utilized in concert to give predictable results. Cosmetic rhinoplasty remains one of the most challenging facial cosmetic procedures. This is unlikely to change despite many advances and changes in this field. The last two decades have witnessed significant contributions to the field of rhinoplasty and have changed both the technical and the philosophical aspects of this surgery. Many of these changes are designed to provide more predictable,

lasting, and enhanced cosmetic results of surgery without compromise of function.

Oral and maxillofacial surgeons have a unique training with extensive and expanding focus on many aspects of the face, including moving the maxilla in three dimensions, repairing frontal, orbital, nasal, or zygomatic fractures, and treating benign and malignant tumors. Although currently not all graduating oral and maxillofacial surgery (OMS) residents are fully exposed to facial cosmetic surgery, it is only logical that cosmetic rhinoplasty, along with other facial esthetic procedures, should be an integral aspect of OMS. This is particularly true because OMS training is so dedicated to all aspects of the facial skeleton and the American Board of OMS tests all candidates in facial cosmetic surgery and expects a certain level of knowledge. We also believe that a majority of training in cosmetic surgery is acquired beyond the residency years. Especially important in cosmetic surgery is the learned benefits of observing over time the results of one's own surgical residency. Rhinoplasty should be thought of as a lifelong learning process due to its complexity.

EDITORS' PERSPECTIVE ON FUTURE RHINOPLASTY

Rhinoplasty, like many other cosmetic procedures, is challenging not only for technical reasons but also because the patient seeking cosmetic surgery often expects an "exceptional" outcome. Unfortunately,

Oral Maxillofacial Surg Clin N Am 24 (2012) ix–x
doi:10.1016/j.coms.2011.11.004

none of the three residency specialties teaching rhinoplasty—oral and maxillofacial surgery, otolaryngology, and plastic surgery—do an "exceptional" job of teaching the surgical resident all the nuances of rhinoplasty. This is why advanced training and continued education in the field of rhinoplasty and cosmetic surgery following one's residency is essential to master this truly challenging field. Surgical "superspecialty" fellowships are becoming more of the norm to immerse the training fellow totally in principles, techniques, and case volumes high enough to give maximum training, experience, and education in this demanding field.

The goal of this issue of *Oral and Maxillofacial Surgery Clinics of North America* is to familiarize the reader with the most current principles of diagnosis and treatment of the rhinoplasty patient as it relates to our specialty. It is not intended as a comprehensive review of the subject, but rather to highlight the important topics, challenges, principles, current thinking, and variations in rhinoplasty surgery. We also hope to stimulate young

surgeons to seek out further training and stimulate research and writing within this field.

Shahrokh C. Bagheri, DMD, MD
Georgia Oral and Facial Surgery, and
Eastern Surgical Associates and Consultants
1880 West Oak Parkway, Suite 215
Marietta, GA 30062, USA

Husain Ali Khan, MD, DMD
Eastern Surgical Associates and Consultants
2795 Peachtree Road NE #2008
Atlanta, GA 30305, USA

Angelo Cuzalina, MD, DDS
7322 East 91 Street South
Tulsa, OK 74133, USA

E-mail addresses:
sbagher@hotmail.com (S.C. Bagheri)
husainakmd@yahoo.com (H.A. Khan)
angelo@tulsasurgicalarts.com (A. Cuzalina)

History of Rhinoplasty

Louis S. Belinfante, DDS

KEYWORDS

- Rhinoplasty • Endonasal approach • External approach
- Free grafting approach • Cosmetic surgery

The word rhinoplasty is derived from 2 Greek words, rhino, meaning nose, and plasikos, meaning to shape or mold.

Since the beginning of recorded time, man has considered the nose to be a key feature, if not the key feature, of facial appearance, beauty, and dynamics. However, because of its central facial location and weak cartilaginous support, the nose is relatively susceptible to disfiguring infection, trauma, pathologic entities, and human-associated carnage. If a person were to be so afflicted, these potential deformities could impose serious alterations to work, social life and psyche. In fact, because the nose has been considered the "organ of reputation," the purposeful amputation of the nose, rhinokopia, was, and is, meant to strip a person of his or her personal honor.[1,2]

IN THE BEGINNING

A papyrus is an ancient form of paper made from the papyrus plant that grows wild in the marshes of the Nile River. The first historical annotation regarding the surgical treatment of nasal deformities is cited in a papyrus named after Edwin Smith. Smith, an American Egyptologist, bought the papyrus from a dealer in Luxor, Egypt, in 1862. The document dates back to approximately 3000 BCE. Dimensions of the papyrus measured 4.68 m long and 33 cm wide, and was divided into 17 pages.

The first transliteration of the papyrus was made by James Henry Breasted in 1930. The papyrus was translated a second time in 2006 by James P. Allen, who was the then curator of Egyptian Art at the Metropolitan Museum of Art in New York, using a more modern understanding of surgical verbiage. Forty-eight surgical cases were discussed beginning at the top of the cranium and ending in the spinal column.[3–5]

At times, the treatment of nasal structural mutilation was surgically attempted by using rudimentary bronze instrumentation. Mutilation was a punishment meted out for major civil offenses, for example, wives leaving the house without permission, adultery, and theft; even lack of female sexual response could lead to punishment causing the recipient visible and lasting humiliation. Captured enemies sometimes were made to suffer the same ill fate as a warning to other would-be adversaries. The treatment of medical problems involved the use of plugs, swabs, linen, and tampons. Strips of adhesive plaster were used for drawing together wound edges. More serious wounds were closed with needles made of materials such as bone, silver, and copper. Surgical sutures were fabricated from plant fibers, hair, or linen. Nasal fractures were treated with stiff rolls of linen.

Other informational pieces concerning nasal deformities were addressed in the Nuzi Tablets (1600–1350 BCE), which originated in the ancient area of Nuzi, 10 miles southwest of the city of Kirkuk in modern Iraq.[6]

The Ebers Papyrus, which is the largest of the medical papyruses and is written in hieratic, devotes an entire section to nasal deformities and their correction. The Ebers Papyrus was also bought by Edwin Smith from an unknown source but was sold early on to Georg Ebers, a German Egyptologist. The papyrus measures 20 m long and has 110 pages. It is dated at 1534 BCE, but parts may have been copied from earlier texts dating back as far as 3400 BCE.[5]

At approximately the same period of time, and as an extremely dynamic, historically significant corollary, one must note with considerable respect the fifth century BCE Ayurvedic physician, Sushruta, who lived around the same period. Although born of a lowly priestly class, the Koomas (potters), he became a professor of medicine at

Dawsonville, GA, USA
E-mail address: Lsbjgb@aol.com

Oral Maxillofacial Surg Clin N Am 24 (2012) 1–9
doi:10.1016/j.coms.2011.10.002

the University of Benares. Within his series of texts, *Sushruta Samhita*, written in Sanskrit (a historical branch of Indo-European languages), he outlined several surgical procedures (300) and described several surgical instruments (121). However, because his writings were in Sanskrit, and the Egyptian writings were in hieroglyphics, the spread of shared medical knowledge was greatly mitigated because of expansive geographic communicative areas. In addition, there was a limited amount of commerce between the areas, even though Alexander the Great from Macedonia in Northern Greece invaded India in 327 BCE. However, his troops lasted there for less than 10 years.

Since purposeful facial deformation was not exclusive to the area of the Fertile Crescent, in India also, there was much opportunity for interested physicians to attempt to repair several contemporaneous facial mutilations. One of the most famous repairs that is associated with Sushruta is the surgical correction of cutoff noses by the transfer of pedicled forehead or cheek flaps to the nasal deformity.[3] Sushruta is also credited with many other surgical procedures, such as those associated with the treatment of cataracts, hernias, lithotomy, and cesarean sections.[7–9]

Nasal disfigurement was used not only on people who made up the average populace but also on societal members of prominent standing. Emperor Justinian II of the Byzantine Empire (circa 700) was overthrown and had his nose mutilated (rhinokopia) and his tongue slit open (glossotomia). The mutilation was performed in front of thousands of cheering former subjects in the middle of the Hippodrome, the sporting and social center of Constantinople, itself, the capital of the Byzantine Empire. The purpose of the mutilation of his nose and tongue was to permanently discourage him from future attempts to regain his throne as emperor. However, after nasal reconstruction, in the Indian manner, and a healed tongue, he was able to return to power. The effects of the mutilation and repair may be noted in his Carmagnola marble statue likeness.[10]

In the first century AD, Rome became a medical center. Two outstanding physicians who lived in Rome and discussed tissue transplantation and treatment of facial defects were Celsus and Galen. Interestingly enough, both physicians were Greek.[11–13]

THE ERA OF DARKNESS

Up to this time, only *reconstructive* nasal surgery was performed. This concept was carried through the Medieval age and up to the Renaissance periods. Very little, if any, surgery to improve appearance was performed during the Dark Ages (fifth to fifteenth centuries).[4]

In 1163, Pope Innocent III and the Council of Tours proclaimed that surgery was to be abandoned by the schools of medicine and all decent physicians. The church believed that surgery was interfering with God's plan.[5] In fact, the performance of a surgical procedure (deemed a manual operation) by an educated physician was considered below his dignity. However, surgical procedures were being performed surreptitiously and were being kept alive by passing on the principles from generation to generation and from one civilization to the next. In this manner, the status quo was maintained but not advanced to any meaningful degree.

In 1442, an Italian surgeon from Sicily named Branca de'Branca introduced a method of using forehead and cheek flaps for facial reconstruction. His son Antonius modified the technique by using the arm as the primary donor site and delaying the initial transfer of the graft. The technique became known as the Italian method. But because of the potential for severe church reprisals, the surgeries that were performed were veiled in secrecy with no publications or even collegial comments.[5]

Pfalzpaint (1450), a German surgeon, described the suture of a biceps flap to the face, which was initially held in position with bandages for several days before the pedicle was separated to form the nasal dorsum.[4]

Gasparo Tagliacozzi (1546–1599) was an Italian surgeon and anatomy professor from Bologna. During this "dark intellectual era" when emphasis was placed on the mundane, he produced scientific writings about his surgical treatments and was given the most credit for the arm flap to the facial area procedures. His fame was great, and after his death, the city fathers of Bologna erected a statue holding a rose in his honor, which symbolized his artistic surgical endeavors. However, dogmatists in the contemporaneous prevailing religious faction had him excommunicated. They thought that Tagliacozzi was "imperiously interfering with the handiwork of God." The religious faction even exhumed his body from a hallowed church burial site and reinterred him in unconsecrated grounds. For the next 2 centuries there was very little advancement in the field of rhinoplasty.[5]

THE REAWAKENING PERIOD

In 1794, B. Lucas, an English surgeon who was working in India reported to have witnessed the reconstruction of a cutoff nose by using a pedicled forehead flap. The operation was performed by a man from the caste of the tile and brick makers in Poona, near the Indian coast. Lucas sent a letter regarding the operation to the *Gentleman's Magazine* of London for the October edition. The account was read by Joseph Carpue, a British surgeon at York Hospital in Chelsea, England. Carpue was piqued by the concept and practiced the procedure on cadavers for approximately 20 years. Finally in 1814, he performed nasal reconstructions on 2 patients. He published the cases in an illustrated monograph where it gained great recognition among European surgeons. Interestingly enough, though Carpue was elected as a Fellow to the Royal College of Surgeons, he was passed over by the same Royal College to sit on their Council. He was disdained by his own contemporaneous professional colleagues.[4,5]

Carl Ferdinand Von Graefe in 1818 published his famous work, *Rhinoplastik*. It had 208 pages and 55 citations. Although he was born in Warsaw, he was educated in Germany and was considered German. In his book, he noted 3 different surgeries: the Indian technique with the forehead flap; the delayed Italian method of Tagliacozzi; and the third, he called the German method that entailed a free graft from the arm. In addition to his rhinoplastic work, he wrote original articles on such subjects as blepharoplasty and cleft palate repair. To many, he is considered the founder of modern plastic surgery. His son became the leading ophthalmologist in Europe. In 1840, Von Graefe, the father, died while performing an operation.[4,5]

Johann Friedrich Dieffenbach succeeded Von Graefe in Berlin with his professorial titles. Dieffenbach was one of the first surgeons to use local anesthesia, and at a later date, ether anesthesia, while performing his rhinoplastic techniques. His book, *Operative Surgery* (1845), discusses nasal reconstruction for over 100 pages. He also discussed the endonasal or the subcutaneous approach to nasal surgery. Some consider him the greatest plastic surgeon of his era.[4,5]

Nasal reconstruction was first performed in the United States by Dr J.M. Warren in Boston, Massachusetts, in the late 1830s. He had previously visited Von Graefe. Dr Warren was related to John Collins Warren, also of Boston. It was the latter Warren who painlessly removed a tumor on a patient's neck with the aid of ether anesthesia administered by William Thomas Green Morton, a dentist, at the Massachusetts General Hospital on October 6, 1846. Morton said to Warren, after administering the ether general anesthetic to the proper surgical depth, his famous words, "Doctor, your patient is ready." On finishing the procedure,

Warren expounded to the surgical attendees present, with his also famous remark about Morton's ether anesthetic, "Gentlemen, this is no humbug."[9,10]

Concurrently and fortuitously, 2 additional discoveries were made that had great impact in broadening the interests of both the surgical and lay communities with regard to the functional and aesthetic advancement of rhinoplastic procedures. They were the discovery of the antiseptic qualities of carbolic acid (phenol) by an English surgeon and the local anesthetic qualities of cocaine.

Joseph Lister in 1867 published his seminal and patient-altering paper on antiseptic principles to reduce infection. The paper was based on the concepts of Louis Pasteur. Lister found that the use of carbolic acid (phenol) greatly mitigated wound infection. As a professor of surgery at the University of Glasgow, he instructed surgeons under his charge to wash their hands before and after operations with a 5% carbolic acid solution and to wear clean gloves. Instruments and the operating theater were sprayed with the same solution. The rate of hospital infections dramatically dropped.[14]

In 1455, the Spanish explorer Augustin de Zarate discovered Peruvian coca. However, it wasn't until approximately 400 years later (1884) that Spanish soldiers while in South America as conquistadors became familiar with the native use of the coca leaf. When brought back to Europe, it was chemically refined into cocaine, which had local anesthetic properties.[15]

One could readily conjecture that an operative procedure that increased the aesthetic value of the face, was relatively comfortable and free of pain for the patient, and in addition, greatly mitigated the chances of infection might gain a potential universal audience. And so it did!

In 1875, William Adams, a dentist, published an article on nasal fracture reduction. He divided the fractures into those associated with bone and those associated with cartilage. Although for one of his patients, initial treatment was initiated at 6 years postfracture, his treatment was earlier and more aggressive than most in an effort to avoid potential fracture-related traumatic deformities. He also fashioned forceps to reduce the fractures that are not unlike those that are still in use today. His concept of external support is also contemporaneous.[16]

Dr John Orlando Roe (1848–1915) was an otolaryngologist from Rochester, New York. In 1887, he published an article regarding a "pug nose." (A pug nose is one with large lower lateral cartilages plus or minus a concavity of the dorsum.) He performed the surgery for purely *aesthetic* reasons, a literature first. Besides, he performed the surgery from an *intranasal approach*, also a first.

However, within the same article, Roe divided the nose into 5 main morphologic classes. One of the classifications was flagrantly anti-Semitic with regard to its implications and the manner in which it was further defined. This classification was probably based on the notations of Robert Knox, a period physiognomist. (For the reader, physiognomy has no scientific basis.)[17-20]

Four years later, in 1891, Roe published a second seminal paper on the correction of angular nasal deformities with great emphasis on the subcutaneous approach. (Dieffenbach, however, is given credit for first introducing the endonasal approach in 1845.) In addition to working from the interior of the nose, he routinely used external and internal splints to keep his postoperative results in their best aesthetic position. Also, he was one of the first to use presurgical and postsurgical photographs to illustrate his results. Some call him the true father of aesthetic rhinoplasty.

Dr Robert F. Weir (1838–1927) is associated with several innovations and modifications in the performance of nasal surgery. For example, he altered Adam's forceps to make them thinner and more delicate for the reduction of fractures. In what he termed an "osteoplastic operation," he used an osteotome to make his fracture reductions "more even." He used osteotomes and forceps to divide the nasal bones in the midline. He also infractured them at their juncture with the maxillae to narrow bone width along with simultaneous elevation of the bony dorsum. However, Weir is probably best known for his attempts to correct nasal dorsum deformities. He inserted the sternum of a freshly killed duck to augment a saddle nose. In retrospect, as one might expect, the heterogeneous graft lasted but a few weeks. His use of a platinum strut was somewhat more successful.[21,22] However, it was James Israel, who in 1896 successfully augmented the saddle nose with a tibial graft.[23] Weir innovatively removed a wedge of the lower lateral cartilages at their facial angle to reduce interalar width and thus created a greater morphologic symmetry. The latter operation is still widely used and bears his name.

ALONG COMES THE WUNDERKIND

Dr Jacques Lewin Joseph (1865–1934) was born and grew up in Königsberg, Prussia (now, Kaliningrad, Russia). He obtained his doctorate in medicine in 1890 at the University of Leipzig, practiced in Berlin for a short period of time, and then studied orthopedic surgery at the J. Wolff Clinic in Berlin. He published his first article on reduction rhinoplasty using an external approach. He later acknowledged that Roe, Weir, and Dieffenbach had preceded him with similar work.

Although Joseph performed plastic procedures on other parts of the body, he is most recognized for devising nasal operations and designing inventive new instruments, which he used to achieve his techno-anatomic goals.

Joseph developed a great ability to conceptualize a reshaped anatomically deficient entity and the biomechanical approach to achieve his well-thought-out goals. As an orthopedist, and for his era, he understood how to transplant osseous tissue like bone from the tibia to the dorsum to correct saddle nose deformities. He studied and classified several nasal deformities and devised individualized procedures for their correction on a scientific basis (unlike physiognomy). His artistic drawings and meticulous operative details definitively established him as a rhinoplastic surgeon par excellence. Later, he insisted that photographs and plaster molds be taken for every patient.

Joseph developed a great many instruments to use for various facets of his devised corrective procedures. For example, for rhinoplasty, he designed various saws to reduce nasal bony and cartilaginous hypertrophies and to have greater control over the lineal separation of lateral nasal fractures for width reduction. He also designed special scalpels for cartilage modification to increase aesthetic contour, external nasal splints, and headbands to hold repaired deviated septa in place. Although Dieffenbach, Roe, and Weir first discussed changes from a subcutaneous approach, it was Joseph, who for years taught and wrote scientific articles concerning the aesthetic reduction and augmentation involving rhinoplastic procedures. Even today, many people believe that most rhinoplastic operations are just variations of Joseph's body of work. One might say that rhinoplasty was born "fully grown" with the emergence of his scientific articles and books.

Joseph died under enigmatic circumstances, while fleeing Hitler's Nazi Germany, in Czechoslovakia in 1934.[5,24-32]

Some who attended Joseph's courses or were contemporaneous with Joseph or his pupils were such great historical names as Gustave Aufricht,[33] Joseph Safian,[34] Jacques Maliniac,[35] John M. Converse,[36] Abe Silver (Silver WE, Abe Silver, personal communication, 2010), and Sam Foman,[37] who in turn gave courses that included Maurice Cottle[38] and Irving Goldman.[39]

It has also been said that Joseph was a bit quirky. During one of his courses, his instruments were placed on an operating room table that was completely covered with a towel so that no one could discern their design. He operated gloveless. Instruments were passed to him covertly from under the towel. One night while taking one of Joseph's courses, Foman persuaded one of Joseph's assistants to show him his instruments. And with lightning speed, Foman drew them all. When Foman returned to the United States, he had a friend from the Klink instrument company manufacture the instruments. He later sold them at his rhinoplasty courses (Silver WE, Sam Foman, personal communication, 2010).[40]

Cottle and Goldman, in due course, gave their own rhinoplastic courses that influenced hundreds of future rhinoplastic surgeons. Many of these gifted surgeons created alterations and some newer rhinoplastic procedures (dome division, elevation of the upper lateral cartilages, additional instrumentation, greater aesthetic forehead flaps, improved postoperative splint dressings, and many other modifications). However, the basic concept came to them, 'fully grown'.

In addition, one cannot exclude other such names as Sir Harold Gillies,[40] V.H. Kazanjian,[41] D.R. Millard,[42] and J.E. Sheehan.[43]

A MAJOR REASSESSMENT

For some surgeons, the endonasal approach had shortcomings. For example, in most instances, surgeons knew from their own formal education, or through observation of other surgeries, researched articles, and case repetitions the subcutaneous disproportionate anatomic morphology of nasal deformities. However, by not being able to directly visualize a problem in situ, the ability to intensely comprehend the anatomic nature of the problem and then treat was compromised. For example, as much subcutaneous fatty and connective tissues (the so-called superficial musculoaponeurotic system layer) as possible might not be removed from above a surgerized dome because of lack of total visualization. This, in turn, might compromise the amount of the final aesthetic acuteness of clarity and shape of tip bulbosity. Thus, a great result might have been diminished to a good result.

Another example might be a visualized actual comparison of the reduction right and left lower lateral cartilages after surgery, but before closure, relative to height, width, symmetry, convexity, and so on.

On a similar note, Ellsworth Toohey once said in Ayn Rand's *The Fountainhead*, "The enemy of excellence is good."[44] Good is not what we want.

Then, in 1970, in Zagreb, in the former Yugoslavia, at a meeting of the American Academy of Facial Plastic and Reconstructive Surgery,[45] a modestly known Yugoslavian surgeon, Ivo F. Padovan, from the meeting city itself, presented a paper on the "The external approach to rhinoplasty."[46] His 10-minute presentation was based on 400 of his own cases and 500 cases of his mentor, Ante Sercer.[47] Both their observations were based on the work of Aurel Rethi of Budapest.[48]

An attendee at the meeting, Dr Robert Simons noted, "A revolutionary shot in the rhinoplasty world had been fired, but it was neither heard nor appreciated immediately."[49]

However, William Goodman, from Toronto, Canada, who was also in attendance at Padovan's lecture, returned home to begin performing the "external approach" for several nasal deformities. He refined the "gull-wing" incision with a resultant greater patient acceptance. Goodman published several articles regarding the positive, aesthetic, and structural outcomes that he was achieving.[50–52]

As fate would have it, at around the same time, a young Canadian otorhinolaryngologist, Peter Adamson, who was very much in tune with Goodman's external approach, began a facial plastic fellowship with Jack Anderson of New Orleans. During this time, Anderson had a renowned reputation for being one of the best known and most well-respected facial plastic surgeons with an unquenchable fire in his belly for the art of rhinoplastic surgery. In addition to these qualities, he was also considered to be a great teacher.[53]

Before the Adamson fellowship, Anderson thought that he could do basically anything endonasally that one could do via an open method. He was very passionate about nasal surgery but was not afraid to try something different if he thought it was biologically just. His practice associate at the time was Calvin Johnson, a well-known facial plastic surgeon in his own right. With Adamson's history with William Goodman and Anderson's scientific inquisitiveness, they started performing external approach rhinoplasties using the midcolumellar approach. In an assessment paper on open rhinoplasty, Anderson, Johnson, and Adamson performed several hundred open procedures, and one of their significant conclusions was that they could not find fault with any surgeon who chose to perform all of their rhinoplasties via the open approach.[54,55]

There have been several alterations in the procedure but nothing that has altered the basic rhinoplastic surgery as postulated by Joseph. Newer alloplastic materials have been used in augmentation settings.[56] Some new instrumentation was developed that made the shaping of cartilage and osseous contouring more effective. However, it is of interest to note, that one of the most inventive rhinoplastic instrument designers who also wrote and lectured on rhinoplastic surgery was a general medical practitioner and not a surgeon per se.[57–59]

Rhinoplasty has come a long way, and along the way many people have benefited from the many surgeons from antiquity to the present. These surgeons have tried to give their patients a more attractive face by altering the one physical anatomic structure that one usually notices first.

NOW COMES ORAL AND MAXILLOFACIAL SURGERY

And with this wonderful circuitous medical history, how did oral and maxillofacial surgery, a dentally based specialty, become a player?

During the early part of the 1980s, after regular American Association of Oral and Maxillofacial Surgeons (AAOMS) board meetings, evening blue sky sessions occurred, involving board and staff members. Nagging questions continued to arise relative to just what was our surgical scope. Had we reached our zenith? Was our surgical breadth already defined and finalized by us or, even worse, by others.

Concurrently, at annual and midwinter meetings, orthognathic surgery programs were almost always assured that lecture halls would be filled to capacity.

The expanded version of orthognathic surgery (or orthodontic surgery as it was then called) was developed to a great degree by European colleagues during the post–World War II era because of a lack of orthodontists and orthodontic materials. Since they could not consistently rely on orthodontic care to aid in the treatment of the many orofacial skeletal deformities, they ingeniously devised technical intraoral methods to operate simultaneously on both the maxillae, the mandible, and their segmental components. Later, definitive biologic credence for these procedures was established by Bell and Levy in 1970 with rhesus monkey angiographic studies.[60] Therefore, it was obvious that facial aesthetics in the form of facial bone reconstruction was paramount in the minds of several members of the orthognathic surgical community.

Serendipitously, for some, pieces of an arcane puzzle started to swirl about during this period. The author's own awareness started when a 17-year-old patient was seen for facial aesthetic evaluation. The patient had recently had orthodontic treatment that involved 4 first bicuspid extractions. If one were to evaluate her postorthodontic models alone, the tooth alignment and achieved occlusion were excellent. However, if one assayed the face, in

its entirety, it became obvious that the lower one-third of the face was severely "dished." As oral and maxillofacial surgeons (OMS), we are well aware that a potential treatment of bimaxillary horizontal retrusion is maxillary and mandibular advancement surgery. This surgery is usually accompanied with a genioplasty.

The concept was presented to the patient's family, and the surgeries were successfully performed. Although the osteotomy sites began to heal in their normal manner and the facial edema subsided, to even a casual observer the patient's previously veiled nasal deformity became the focal point of her face. The patient's family sought the services of a rhinoplastic surgeon. The surgery was performed and I saw the patient several weeks later. She had become a swan! I was stunned. I thought that out of all the facial surgeries recently performed on her, the nasal alterations made, by far, the greatest significant impact in her overall facial aesthetics.

Although, at the time OMS were performing rhinoplasties to only the slightest moderate degree, the thought occurred that as OMS, we operate lateral to the nose, inferior to the nose, above the nose, and on occasion, within the nose. Why should we not perform aesthetic operations on the nose in combination with other facial procedures, or as a stand-alone procedure? After all, we are OMS. And the nose is clearly in the center of the maxillofacial region. Why not?

But who would teach an oral surgeon, and better yet, one without a medical degree? Enter, Dr William (Billy) Silver, an otolaryngologist by formal post–medical school residency training. After living in the same area for several years, Dr Silver and I had become geographic friends who shared ideas, techniques, generalized information, and stories about people and events in our respective specialties.

Dr Silver's brother was an orthodontist, his father, a general dentist, and his uncle, Abe Silver, a rhinoplastic surgeon. His uncle, Abe, was part of New York's well-known Mount Sinai Hospital's rhinoplastic teaching group along with Irving Goldman. Dr Goldman was the creator of the famous nasal dome division for greater tip definition, which bears his name (the Goldman tip).

Dr Billy Silver received additional training after his formal otorhinolaryngology residency by spending much time with Drs Richard Webster of Boston, Jack Anderson of New Orleans, and Maury Parks of Los Angeles. This was the route taken by many future facial plastic surgeons even before there was an official subspecialty of facial plastic surgery and, for that matter, facial plastic fellowships. These members were indeed the pioneers of this new specialty. It was not an easy row to hoe logistically, politically, or financially for these potential members of the newest specialty in the head and neck region. There was a great deal of opposition to the formation of the specialty from anatomically regional medical competitors.[61] In fact, $1.2 million was levied in a lawsuit that weighed against the Georgia Society of Plastic Surgeons regarding the professional competency of facial plastic surgeons.[62,63]

With this background in mind, a telephone call was made to Dr Billy Silver. When asked if he were sitting down, his answer was yes. "Billy, I would like you to teach me how to do rhinoplasties." There was a pause on the phone, which seemed to me like 1 hour but was actually just momentary. I thought he had fallen off the chair, fainted, or both. At the end of this pregnant pause, he answered with resolve in his voice stating that he would be more than delighted to teach me. He mentioned a book that he wanted me to read.[64] He also asked me to call his receptionist for a list of rhinoplasties that he had scheduled so I could initially observe the mechanics and instrumentation.

And so it began. To say the least, it was exciting! I spent time with him that year and with other surgeons, while also attending several meetings.[65] The 1988 AAOMS Midwinter meeting on the topic of *Esthetic Considerations in Oral and Maxillofacial Surgery* held in Tucson, not an easy place to get to, was up to that time the largest midwinter meeting ever attended. The topics included liposuction, facial augmentation, rhinoplasty, cheiloplasty, and others.

The American Academy of Cosmetic Surgery was a fledgling organization devoted to cosmetic surgery. The academy consisted of a group of professionals in search of a platform to share and add to their cosmetic knowledge. I attended a few meetings and then submitted the required number of cases to become a full member. They were good to OMS. Academy presidents such as Julius Newman, Howard Tobin, and Tom Alt opened their offices to academy members for the observation of patient treatment. Their only criterion was an interest in cosmetic surgery. It was also there that I had the privilege of meeting Richard Webster while I was a member of the academy board. It was his philosophy that every specialty brings something unique to the cosmetic surgery table. Early on, for the OMS who was interested in performing cosmetic surgery, the academy was like a home away from home, but never forgetting that home was truly the AAOMS.

Some books on rhinoplasty were somewhat confusing to me until I read *Open Structure Rhinoplasty* by Calvin Johnson and Dean Toriumi.[66] The book was transforming. I read it, reread it, made

flash cards, and then I was fortunate to spend a week in Dr Johnson's office. Sheen's 2-volume text is also a giant in the rhinoplastic literature.[67] After about a year, I started to perform rhinoplastic procedures myself. First, dorsal hump removals and gradually into the more intricate dome and lateral osteotomies. These were performed, at first with orthognathic surgeries and later as stand-alone procedures. Over a period of time, but gradually, the local hospital staff credentialing committees were won over. Patients who formerly underwent rhinoplasty and orthognathic surgery asked if facelifts, eyes, and peels were in our specialties preview. And then the process started all over again.

During this period of time, representatives of the AAOMS met with the American Board of Oral and Maxillofacial Surgery. The 2 national organizations updated the definition of the specialty to include the treatment of facial aesthetic defects. The house of delegates of the American Dental Association later ratified this change. Although some dental

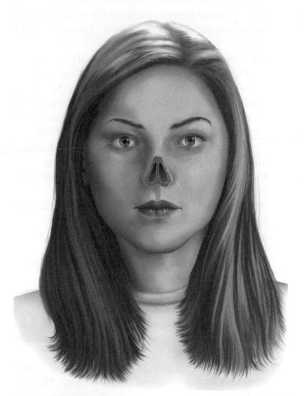

Fig. 1. Sketch of a young, mutilated 18 year-old woman based upon a recent punishment administered to her by her husband and in-laws for not allowing them to continuously subject her to demeaning and abusive behavior.

boards were recalcitrant in accepting the change because of several frivolous reasons, a significant number of individual states changed their definition with rapidity to coincide with the more realistic definitions of our national organizations.

So we can say with assurance, that rhinoplasty and oral and maxillofacial surgery are now tightly interwoven in the future of the specialties scope. And in fact, can any other specialty routinely surgically alter the maxillae, advance it anteriorly, reduce its height, increase its height, alter the mandibular morphology, make it longer or shorter, and so forth? The same could be said for the chin and then a rhinoplasty could be performed to balance out the aesthetics of the face.

And lastly, one can also state that the services of those that also perform reconstructive facial plastic surgery is still a very much needed surgical therapy (**Fig. 1**).

REFERENCES

1. Mc Dowel F. The source book of plastic surgery. Baltimore (MD): Waverly Press; 1977.
2. Tiranic G. The mutilated nose: rhinokopia as a visual mark of sexual offence. Presented at the 29th Annual Byzantine Studies Conference. Lewiston (ME), October 16–19, 2003.
3. Breasted JH. The Edwin Smith Surgical Papyrus, vol. 1. Chicago: University of Chicago; 1930. p. 1–29.
4. Whitaker IS, Karoo RO, Spyrou G, et al. The birth of plastic surgery: the story of nasal reconstruction from the Edwin Smith Papyrus to the twenty-first century. Plast Reconstr Surg 2007;120:327–36.
5. Eisenberg I. A history of rhinoplasty. S Afr Med J 1982;62:286–92.
6. Maltz M. Evolution of plastic surgery. New York: Frorben Press; 1946. p. 27–31.
7. Bhishagratna KK. The Sushruta Samhita (English translation based on the original Sanskrit text). Varanasi (India): Chowkhamba Sanskrit Series Office; 1963.
8. Tewari M, Shukla HS. Sushruta: the father of Indian surgery. Ind J Surg 2005;67(4):229–30.
9. Garrison FH. An introduction to the history of medicine. Philadelphia: WB Saunders; 1917. p. 60–2.
10. Remensnyder JP, Bigelow ME, Goldwyn RM. Justinian II and Carmagnola: a Byzantine rhinoplasty? Plast Reconstr Surg 1979;63:19–20.
11. Foman S. The surgery of injury and plastic repair. Baltimore (MD): Williams and Wilkins; 1939. p. 614–831.
12. Rinzler CA. The encyclopedia of cosmetic and plastic surgery. New York: Facts on File; 2009. p. 150–4.
13. Lipp RL. Medical landmarks USA. New York: McGraw-Hill; 1991. p. 45.
14. Lister J. On the antiseptic principle in the practice of surgery. Br Med J 1867;2(351):245–60.
15. Knapp H. Hydrochlorate of cocaine—experiments and application. Med Rec 1884;26:461.
16. Adams W. On the treatment of broken nose by forcible straightening and mechanical retentive apparatus. Br Med J 1875;2:421.
17. Lam SM. John Orlando Roe: father of aesthetic rhinoplasty. Arch Facial Plast Surg 2002;4:122–3.
18. Roe JO. A classic reprint: the deformity termed "pug-nose" and its correction, by a simple operation. Aesthetic Plast Surg 1986;10:89–91.
19. Roe JO. The correction of angular deformities of the nose by a subcutaneous operation. Med Rec 1891;40(3).
20. Efron J. Defenders of the race. New Haven (CT): Yale University Press; 1994.
21. Weir RF. On the relief of the deformity of a broken nose by some new methods. Med Rec 1880;17:279.
22. Weir RF. On restoring sunken noses without scaring the face. N Y Med J 1892;56:449.
23. Israel J. Two new methods of rhinoplasty. Arch Klin Chir 1896;53:255–8.
24. Joseph J. Operative reduction of the size of a nose (rhinomiosis). Berl Klin Wochenschr 1898;40:882.
25. Joseph J. About some further nasal reductions. Plastic Recon Surg 1971;47:82.
26. Joseph J. Nasal reductions. Dtsch Med Wochenschr 1914;30:1095. Translation published in Plast Reconstr Surg 1971;47:79.
27. Joseph J. Treatise on rhinoplasty. Berl Klin Wochenschr 1907;44:470.
28. Joseph J. Correction of twisted nose. Dtsch Med Wochenschr 1907;49:203.
29. Joseph J. Corrective nasal plastic. In: Katz L, Blumenfeld F, editors. Handbuch der Speziellen Chirurgie. Leipzig (Germany): C Kabitsch; 1922.
30. Joseph J. Nasal plastic and various face plastics, as well as mammoplasty. Leipzig (Germany): C Kabitsch; 1931.
31. Swanepoel PF, Eisenberg I. Current concepts in cosmetic rhinoplasty. S Afr Med J 1981;60:536–44.
32. Mc Dowell F. History of rhinoplasty. Aesthetic Plast Surg 1978;1:321–48.
33. Aufricht G. Hints and surgical details in rhinoplasty. Laryngoscope 1943;53:317.
34. Safian J. Corrective rhinoplastic surgery. New York: Paul Hoeber Co; 1935.
35. Maliniac JW. Procedure for elevation of nasal dorsum by transposition of lateral cartilages. Arch Otolaryngol 1945;41:214.
36. Converse JM. Corrective surgery of nasal deviations. Arch Otolaryngol 1950;52:5.
37. Foman S. Physiologic principles of rhinoplasty. Arch Otolaryngol 1951;53:3.
38. Barelli PT. Maurice H. Cottle, MD. Otolaryngol Head Neck Surg 1944;110(6):482–6.

39. Goldman IB. The importance of the medial crura in nasal tip reconstruction. Arch Otolaryngol 1957;65: 143–7.
40. Gilles H. Plastic surgery of the face. Theime-Stratton Coerp. Expanded Edition; 1983.
41. Kazanjian VH. Nasal deformities of syphilitic origin. Plast Reconstr Surg 1948;3:517.
42. Millard DR Jr. Alar margin sculpturing. Plast Reconstr Surg 1967;40:337.
43. Sheehan JE. Plastic surgery of the nose. 1st edition. New York: Paul Haber Co; 1978. p. 19.
44. Rand A. The fountainhead. Bobbs-Merill Co; 1943.
45. American Academy of Facial Plastic Surgery and Reconstructive Surgery. Od Proceedings of the First International Symposium of the AAFPRS New York. New York: Grune & Stratton; 1972.
46. Padovan L. External approach to rhinoplasty (decortication). Symp ORL Jug 1960;3–4:354–60.
47. Sercer A, Mundnich K. Plastiche Operationen an der Ohrmuschel. Stuttgart (Germany): Georg. Thieme Verlag; 1962.
48. Rethi AC. Operation to shorten an excessively long nose. Der Chirurg 1929;1:1103–5.
49. Simon R. Perspectives on the evolution of rhinoplasty. Arch Facial Plast Surg 2009;2:409–11.
50. Goodman WS. External approach to rhinoplasty. Can J Otolaryngol 1973;2:207–10.
51. Goodman WS, Charbonneau PA. External approach to rhinoplasty. Laryngoscope 1974;84:2195–201.
52. Goodman WS, Charles PA. Technique of external rhinoplasty. Can J Otolaryngol 1978;7:9–12.
53. Sepehr A, Adamson P. The legacy of Jack Anderson. Arch Fac Plas Surg 2009;11(6):412–3.
54. Anderson JR, Johnson CM, Adamson P. Open rhinoplasty: an assessment. Otolaryngol Head Neck Surg 1982;90:272–4.
55. Anderson JR, Ries WR. Rhinoplasty: emphasizing the external approach. New York: Thieme, Inc; 1986.
56. Abn MS, Moohian N, Maas CS, et al. Total nasal reconstruction with alloplastic and autogenous grafts. Facial Plast Surg 1998;14:145.
57. Rubin F. Reconstruction of bony nasal pyramid. Arch Otolaryngol 1968;88:77–80.
58. Rubin F. Permanent change in shape of cartilage by morselization. Arch Otolaryngol 1969;89:64–70.
59. Rubin F. Controlled tip sculpturing with the morselizer. Arch Otolaryngol 1983;109:160–3.
60. Bell W, Levy B. Healing after anterior maxillary osteotomy. J Oral Surg 1970;28(10):728–34.
61. Rusca JA, Huger WE. Things are never what they seem, skim milk masquerades as cream. J Med Assoc Ga 1982;71:103–5.
62. Anderson JR. An old specialty puts on a new face … and head … and neck. South Med J 1980;73(8):1058–62.
63. Silver W, Anderson JR. An old medical specialty puts on a new face … and head … and neck. J Med Assoc Ga 1981;70:723–4.
64. Rees T, Baker D, Tabbal N. Rhinoplasty problems and controversies. St Louis (MO): CV Mosby; 1988.
65. Rhinoplasty 88. Meeting of American Academy of Facial Plastic Surgeons. Key Biscayne (FL); Dec 10–15, 1988.
66. Johnson CM, Toriumi DM. Open structure rhinoplasty. Philadelphia: WB Saunders; 1990.
67. Sheen JH. Aesthetic rhinoplasty. St Louis (MO): CV Mosby; 1978.

Rhinoplasty: Initial Consultation and Examination

Husain Ali Khan, MD, DMD

KEYWORDS

- Rhinoplasty • Preoperative consultation • Cosmesis
- Nasal symmetry

ETHNIC, CULTURAL, AND GENDER DIFFERENCES

It is often said that beauty is in the eye of the beholder. However, the perception of beauty is continually evolving. As with fashion, our minds adapt to new trends and our eyes progressively break away from traditional patterns. The public often looks to actors, musicians, sports stars, and politicians to set trends in fashion and beauty.

Not unlike the fashion industry, the trends in cosmetic surgery are continually changing, although the general sentiment of youthful appearance is a common denominator. As cosmetic surgeons, it is extremely important to step out of our personal perceptions of beauty and surgical norms and understand the perspective of the patient. Cosmetic parameters for beauty have regional, ethnic, and cultural differences. The surgeon needs to consider the classic norms that pertain to a patient and must never compromise form for function. A successful cosmetic result with compromise of function is a failure.

When consulting with patients of a specific ethnicity, it is important to determine how much of their ethnicity they wish to preserve. In some cases, the patient may only want to make a minimal change to a particular feature (for example, a large dorsal hump or a wide alar base). A surgeon must quickly understand and be comfortable with the patient's expectations and desires of cosmetic surgery.

Today, cosmetic surgeons treat all segments of the population. In the past, cosmetic surgery was only considered to be fashionable by wealthy female patients. Current cosmetic surgery encompasses all socioeconomic classes and genders. In fact, younger patients and male patients are increasingly interested in cosmetic surgery.

In addition to surgical and dermatologic cosmetic procedures, the surgeon should be an advocate of general preventive health care. The cosmetic and rhinoplasty consultation allows the opportunity to assess overall wellness, and it is the author's opinion that performing cosmetic surgery on a patient who is not involved in an appropriate wellness program or does not make an active effort to improve his or her overall health may be counterproductive. Nutrition, exercise, and a healthy lifestyle are the foundations of successful cosmetic surgical interventions. Good nutrition and exercise optimizes a person's cardiovascular system and improves cellular turnover. General facial and body appearance often dramatically improve with weight reduction, especially in the younger population. A patient who maintains his or her body mass index within the healthy norms will generally be considered more attractive. In many instances, if overweight patients return to their optimal weight through diet and exercise their appearance will greatly improve, and this will also help the surgeon to determine the extent of the cosmetic defect versus excessive weight. It is important that patients be cautioned that most cosmetic surgical procedures (including body liposuction) are not intended for weight loss.

INITIAL CONSULTATION

Selection of patients is one of the most difficult components of facial cosmetic surgery, and is

Eastern Surgical Associates and Consultants, 2795 Peachtree Road NE #2008, Atlanta, GA 30305, USA
E-mail address: husainakmd@yahoo.com

Oral Maxillofacial Surg Clin N Am 24 (2012) 11–24
doi:10.1016/j.coms.2011.11.002
1042-3699/12/$ – see front matter © 2012 Elsevier Inc. All rights reserved.

especially important for surgeons with less experience. Being able to understand a patient and his or her needs is one of the most important skills a surgeon can have. Occasionally, during an initial encounter with a patient the surgeon may be so excited to have a patient showing interest in having a particular procedure that he or she may forget to determine whether the patient is truly a candidate for cosmetic surgery. The surgeon must be thorough in the initial evaluation to determine whether the patient is psychologically and physically stable enough for surgery.

The interpretation of a patient's desires is the most important factor in determining patient satisfaction. A surgeon can perform a perfect operation; however, if the results do not meet the patient's expectations this will result in an unhappy patient. Such a situation is frequently attributable to the inadequate preoperative interpretation of the patient's desire or to unreasonable expectations that were not recognized. The ultimate goal is for the patient to be happy and for the surgeon to be proud of the work completed.

It is fundamental that during the initial visit, a trusting patient-doctor relationship is established, facilitating the comfort and willingness to express goals and concerns for cosmetic surgery. The patient should be allowed to freely express his or her chief complaint without interruption. The presence of an assistant is highly encouraged. Asking open-ended questions such as "How can I help you?" or "What brings you to see us today?" allows the patient to express needs and concerns. Specific questions such as "Are you here to discuss the bump on your nose?" should be avoided. The examination and the interview process are best done with access to mirrors to allow improved communication regarding facial anatomic regions.

Medical History

As with any other surgical procedure, a thorough medical history is imperative. Conditions that affect wound healing (such as diabetes, autoimmune connective tissue disorders, hepatic and renal insufficiency) need to be managed adequately before committing to surgery. The cardiopulmonary status of the patient for administration of safe general anesthesia should be assessed. Uncontrolled hypertension should be managed preoperatively to avoid unstable swings in blood pressure, and to aid in homeostasis and prevent hematoma formation.

Psychiatric illnesses should be noted and investigated prior to any surgical intervention. The presurgical period is well defined whereas the postsurgical care is "infinite." Therefore, surgeons should use caution with prior or current psychological diagnosis that may compromise results.

The following specific conditions and diagnostic factors are noted.

Patients with unrealistic expectations

These patients may present in two general categories:

1. Patients who present with pictures of celebrities and request that the doctor transforms their face to conform to the image; such patients may bring magazine photographs of models with highlighted features or a particular form they want the surgeon to mimic
2. Patients who request drastic changes that would make the face disproportionate; such patients often seek opinions of multiple surgeons

Obsessive-compulsive personality trait/ obsessive-compulsive disorder

Obsessive-compulsive disorder (OCD) is a specific diagnosis defined in the *Diagnostic and Statistical Manual of Mental Disorders* (Fourth Edition, Text Revised), which is distinguished from obsessive-compulsive personality (OCP) trait. The essential features of OCD are recurrent obsessions or compulsions that are severe enough to be time consuming (ie, they take up more than 1 hour a day), or cause marked distress or significant impairment. OCP traits include common obsessions or compulsions such as: (1) constant, irrational worry about germs, dirt, or contamination; (2) feelings that something bad will happen if certain items are out of order or place; (3) fear that thoughts will cause someone harm; and (4) preoccupation with throwing away or losing items that have little value.

Patients who are perfectionists fall into this category. These patients are usually well dressed and are often overly compulsive when arranging the initial examination. Usually they have been treated by other surgeons, and have complaints about them; they may have a long list of unrealistic questions. These patients magnify any minor imperfections or asymmetry, and demand immediate correction. Perfectionists are, by nature, never happy with themselves and will never be happy with the surgical result.

"Let's do the surgery now" patients

These patients wish the surgeon to perform the surgery immediately, feel no need for a proper evaluation, and put tight time limits on the surgeon. Such patients generally have little patience with the surgeon's efforts to be thorough during the examination, and do not want to hear or care about complications or any possibility of poor surgical outcome. Usually these patients have undergone some previous underlying psychological event.

Doubtful patients
These patients have often had multiple consultations and are unclear about which procedure they wish to undergo. Such patients are uncertain about whether they really want to have a procedure, and often prefer the surgeon to take a paternalistic rather than autonomous approach toward decisions, often stating "do whatever you think is best." Doubtful patients are usually seeking cosmetic surgery following a suggestion of a relative or career advisor. The hallmark of these patients is that they are vague about what would make them happy. Surgery is frequently scheduled, canceled, and rescheduled again.

Patients with rude demeanor
These patients are generally pleasant to the surgeon but when dealing with the office assistants and hospital staff they can be pushy and demeaning, and demand preferential treatment. These unpleasant traits usually surface during the initial evaluation as inappropriate, disagreeable behavior.

Excessively complimentary patients
These patients are generally full of compliments, and praise the surgeon's expertise and reputation. By careful probing the surgeon might determine that the patient has had previous consultations and outcomes that were not satisfactory. These patients often travel great distances to see the surgeon, with little background knowledge of the doctor or practice. Surgeons should therefore be cautious, as such patients can quickly turn on them if the surgical outcome has minor imperfections. The compliments may be turned into anger.

Patients with minor or imagined deformity
At first, most surgeons would agree that a small modification of a minimal deformity might result in a perfect result. However, this may not be the case when dealing with a patient who is overemphasizing a minor deformity. In the mind of such patients a minor deformity is as large as a major deformity. These patients are often seeking perfection, and the surgeon must be very careful not to fall into this trap.

Depression
During the initial evaluation and history, the surgeon must be aware of a history or a present diagnosis of depression. The social history of a patient can determine stability in a patient's life. Facial cosmetic surgery may temporarily improve the mood

of a depressed patient, but does not rid the patient of the underlying cause. An evaluation by a therapist is prudent in these situations.

Body dimorphic disorder
Body dimorphic disorder (BDD) is defined as a preoccupation with an imagined or slight defect in appearance that leads to significant impairment in functioning. Any area of the body may be a center of concern. Some studies show that up to 7% of women who seek cosmetic surgery meet the criteria for BDD. There is 2% prevalence in the general public. Reports have shown that the majority of patients with BDD do not benefit from cosmetic surgery, and in some cases patients have become violent toward themselves or the surgeon. If a surgeon has any suspicions preoperatively that a patient may suffer from BDD, a psychological evaluation may be indicated to rule out BDD.

Eating disorders
Patients with anorexia and bulimia generally have a poor self-image and are underweight, with an altered nutritional status. These patients can be at risk during the perioperative period. Extreme caution has to be taken when screening this type of patient. When dealing with patients with

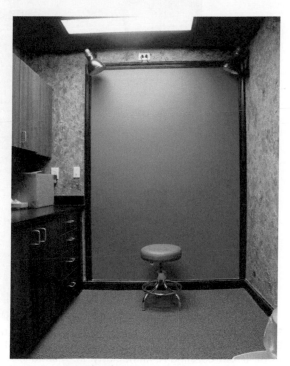

Fig. 1. An example of a photographic setup for a rhinoplasty examination. A simple setup consisting of a camera and a clean background is sufficient; however, a sophisticated system consisting of a standardized lighting, size, and camera settings is beneficial.

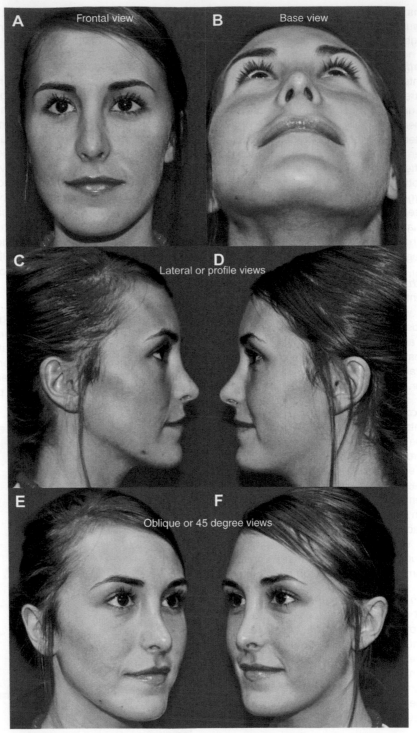

Fig. 2. (*A–F*) The 6 standard views shown should be taken for all rhinoplasty patients before and after surgery. Except for the base view, the patient's head should always have the Frankfort horizontal plane parallel with the floor. (*From* Cuzalina A. Rhinoplasty. In: Niamtu J, editor. Cosmetic facial surgery. St Louis (MO): Elsevier; 2011. p. 175–246; with permission.)

possible eating disorders, an important question is whether they are happy and satisfied with their current weight. Weight fluctuations in some patients can be very noticeable in the face. Significant weight fluctuations can be caused by underlying metabolic or psychological disorders. Red flags should be raised if a patient has lost more than 10 pounds (4.5 kg) in the past year or is constantly changing diets. Some cosmetic surgeons will advise their patients that if they plan to lose more than 10% of their body weight, they should defer surgery until their weight has stabilized. It has been shown that patients who exercise regularly bounce back from surgery much quicker than those who have a sedentary lifestyle. In an aging face, both weight gain and weight loss can give a perception of increased age.

Evaluation of a patient for rhinoplasty involves the establishment of a trusting relationship with the surgeon and interpretation of the patients' expectations. Insufficient preoperative discussions and clarification of patients' expectations has led to a sizable population of unsatisfied patients. The surgeon has to be firm on redirecting or denying surgery for expectations that are unreasonable or surgically unobtainable.

Other issues

Other important factors include the amount of sun exposure, history of sunburn, and the use of sunscreen. Risk factors for skin cancer should be considered. A history of hypertension and blood dyscrasias must be thoroughly investigated. Postoperative hematoma formation after rhinoplasty surgery can present as a septal hematoma, and nasal bleeds from osteotomies can be complications of undiagnosed coagulopathies or prolonged uncontrolled elevated blood pressure. Blood dyscrasias can be discovered through family history, or a history of increased bruising or prolonged bleeding after a dental extraction.

The use of herbal supplementation must be thoroughly investigated, because some constituents may affect the coagulation cascade. Patients at high risk for deep venous thrombosis prophylaxis should be recognized, and appropriate preventive

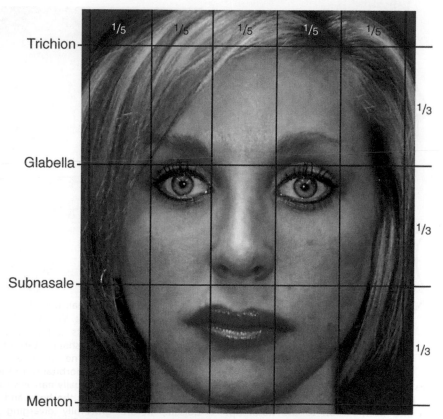

Fig. 3. Nasal and general facial proportion is typically described as depicted here. Achieving harmony from cosmetic surgery often means correcting disproportions. The nose takes up the middle third and middle fifth, and its strategic location makes proper proportion even more critical. (*From* Cuzalina A. Rhinoplasty. In: Niamtu J, editor. Cosmetic facial surgery. St Louis (MO): Elsevier; 2011. p. 175–246; with permission.)

protocols should be followed. The use of potent anti-coagulants such as warfarin and clopidogrel should be discontinued or reduced in conjunction with the primary care or other involved medical specialist. It is also recommended to discontinue aspirin products and nonsteroidal anti-inflammatory drugs, as well as herbal and health supplementation (eg, vitamin E, ginkgo biloba, St John's wort) 2 weeks before the procedure. Isotretinoin should also be discontinued, as this may delay wound healing.

Social History

Numerous studies have shown that poor wound healing and complications with wound healing are associated with smoking. Patients should be educated on the importance of smoking cessation. If complete cessation cannot be achieved, a minimum of 2 weeks with no exposure to tobacco products is warranted. A history of alcohol abuse or dependence should be investigated prior to surgical treatment. In cases where a patient has

undergone a recent traumatic event (loss of job, divorce, loss of a loved one) it may be wise to delay surgery until emotional stability has been achieved.

Surgical History

Prior anesthetic and surgical complications must be investigated. The number of prior cosmetic surgical procedures including revisions should be noted. Patients who have had multiple cosmetic procedures, especially for the same anatomic location, should be handled with extreme caution.

PHYSICAL EXAMINATION

Overall physical examination is imperative for anyone undergoing cosmetic rhinoplasty under general anesthesia or total intravenous anesthesia. The surgeon must also examine the scalp, skull, ears, and chest wall for potential harvest sites for bone and cartilage.

The examination of the patient presenting for cosmetic rhinoplasty surgery takes place after a thorough consultation and determination of the

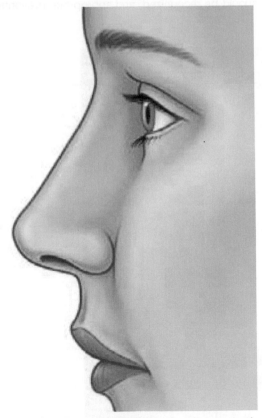

Fig. 4. The dorsum starts from the nasion to tip-defining points. Its contour is relatively straight, 1 to 2 mm below a line from nasion to the nasal tip. (*From* Marin VP, Cochran CS, Gunter JP. Anatomic approach for tip problems. In: Aston SJ, et al, editors. Aesthetic plastic surgery. St Louis (MO): Elsevier; 2009. p. 507–21; with permission.)

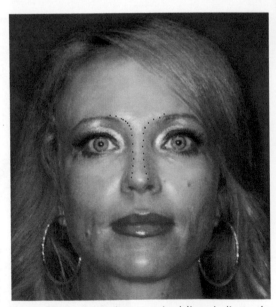

Fig. 5. The red, curvilinear, paired lines indicate the brow-to-tip aesthetic line. When on frontal view, an outline of the highlights cast on the nose should form a subtle hourglass shape. Starting superiorly at the medial brow, the line curves along a concave path following the supraorbital rim to join the radix or nasal root, then gradually narrows to form a relatively straight line along the bony and cartilaginous dorsum, before gracefully diverging outward to outline a slightly wider nasal supratip and fading laterally along a confluent alar-tip lobule. (*Data from* Toriumi DM. New concepts in nasal tip contouring. Arch Facial Plast Surg 2006;8:156–85.)

patient's chief complaints. The author prefers to examine the patient in front of a 3-way mirror. A wall mirror with the aid of a hand-held mirror is also adequate.

Although every surgeon has a different approach, a systematic method that addresses all areas of concern is recommended. The examination also allows the patient to point out areas of interest that may not have been addressed during the consultation. Once the surgeon understands the patient's needs and complaints, he or she can offer recommendations that may achieve the patient's goals. The examination comprises assessment of hard tissue (skeletal features) and structures (frontal bone, zygoma, maxillomandibular complex). The dentition and occlusion is examined for anterior dental aesthetic, evaluation of dentofacial deformities (eg, maxillary hypoplasia/hyperplasia), and angle classification. The soft tissue is examined for signs of laxity and hyperdynamic lines, and fat distribution in the forehead, periorbital areas, midface, mandible, and neck. Finally the skin is assessed for signs of photoaging and general skin health, and absence of pathology.

Examination of the skin peels and laser treatment work better with certain Fitzpatrick types.

Thickness quality and quantity, the amount of mobility, sebaceous glands, and hypopigmentation/hyperpigmentation are important factors to be documented when examining the skin. It is also important to make a note of previous surgical scars, and all suspicious precancerous lesions must be thoroughly investigated.

Following an overall facial cosmetic surgery examination, the surgeon can now focus on a detailed cosmetic rhinoplasty examination.

Photographic Documentation

The photographic setup often differs among surgeons. A simple setup consisting of a camera and a clean background is sufficient; however, a sophisticated system consisting of standardized lighting, size, and camera settings is beneficial. The extent of the photographic setup is determined by the specific needs of the surgeon; however, most cosmetic surgeons find it valuable to invest in high-quality office photography equipment (**Fig. 1**).

It is the author's opinion that photographs should be taken by the surgeon or by a trained assistant to ensure standardization of preoperative and postoperative images. Not only is this

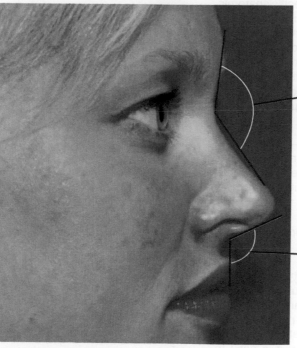

Nasofrontal angle normal 115-130 degrees

Nasolabial angle 95-105 degrees for females, 90-95 degrees for males

Fig. 6. Two common nasal-facial angle measurements are the nasofrontal and nasolabial angles. Achieving angulations within norms for a given patient will help achieve an aesthetically pleasing nose. Abnormalities in angulations and facial proportions appear much worse than minor asymmetries or shape irregularities. The nasofrontal angle is often slightly more obtuse in females. Likewise, the nasolabial angle is ideally more obtuse in females than in males. (*From* Cuzalina A. Rhinoplasty. In: Niamtu J, editor. Cosmetic facial surgery. St Louis (MO): Elsevier; 2011. p. 175–246; with permission.)

valuable when dealing with patients but is also important for academic presentations and for possible publication. The author's standardized set of photos includes 6 views: frontal view, left and right lateral and oblique views (45°), and worm's view or basilar view (which allows the surgeon to visualize the nasal base, alar, and nostrils). Other views that may be obtained include relaxed frontal and high smiling. It is important to have the photographs standardized, especially for viewing with the patient during the 6- to 18-month postoperative course of rhinoplasty (**Fig. 2**).

Overall Nasal Symmetry

The nose must be evaluated overall for symmetry in relation to the face (**Fig. 3**) and also to considerations in gender, age, ethnicity, and overall body habitus. One must understand the basic acceptable norms for each category, which also gives the surgeon another opportunity to understand what the patient finds attractive and what the patient wants. Frequently the patient may desire certain changes that are surgically unrealistic; at this point the surgeon needs to educate the patient as to what can be realistically achieved. It is better for the surgeon to promise less but deliver more.

The nose can be addressed by specific anatomic and functional parameters. The skin, radix, dorsum, tip, nasal base, and nasal airway are used by the author as specific anatomic regions that can be surgically modified for cosmetic improvement. This simplistic approach allows the development of a cosmetic treatment plan for each region that is organized into an overall surgical plan.

The Skin Envelope

In the initial evaluation of the nose, most beginner rhinoplasty surgeons tend to forget to evaluate the skin envelope. Within the different ethnic populations one must recognize the variability between the skin envelopes. In the author's opinion it is one of the most important structures of the nose. The skin must be evaluated for thickness texture, sebaceous content, and pigmentation. There is little fibrofatty tissue in the skin overlying the dorsum; it gradually increases over the tip and is most abundant in the alar region. Most surgeons agree that a middle ground between thick and thin skin is ideal for cosmetic rhinoplasty. In skin that is very thin it is easy to show all the detail of the cartilaginous and bony framework, making it a challenge also to hide imperfections. Thick skin, on the other hand, does not show all the details of the changes that are made to bony and cartilaginous framework;

an example of this can be seen during changes made to the nasal tip, many of which often go unnoticed. The benefit of thick skin is that it hides imperfections of changes and camouflages unpredictable changes as the nasal tip scars over time. Debulking of the underlying flap is useful but limited, due to compromise of the overlying skin with removal of excessive soft tissue.

Dorsum and Radix

The dorsum consists of the osseocartilaginous dorsum to the tip and the interface with the glabella and subnasale. The dorsum can be described by the contour, height, length, and interface angles. The dorsum starts from the nasion (some clinicians argue that the radix is the true take-off point) to tip-defining points. Its contour is relatively straight, 1 to 2 mm below a line from nasion to the nasal tip (**Fig. 4**), and some surgeons believe that the contour should be even more ski-sloped in females.

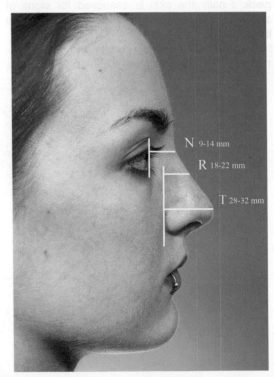

Fig. 7. Measuring nasal height. Nasal height is measured at the nasion (N), rhinion (R), and tip-defining point (T) (pronasalae). The reference of origin for the nasion begins at the anterior corneal plane, whereas the vertical alar plane is referenced when measuring rhinion height and tip projection. Standard averages for each region are shown. (*From* Stelger JD, Baker SR. Nuances of profile management: the radix. Facial Plast Surg Clin North Am 2009;17: 15–28; with permission.)

The rhinion is the point where the bony dorsum and cartilaginous dorsum integrate; it is slightly concave in females and convex in males. In males this can very pronounced, especially in certain ethnic groups.

The frontal-view brow-tip aesthetic line is a continuous curvilinear line extending from the medial brow to the nasal tip (**Fig. 5**). As outlined in **Fig. 4**, the narrowest portion is along the nasal vault, and the line diverges laterally both superiorly toward the brow and inferiorly to the nasal tip. The inclination of the lateral walls is roughly 57°. The skin overlying the dorsum is thickest at the radix and thinnest over the rhinion. The ideal width of the aesthetic line is 6 to 8 mm in females and 8 to 10 mm in males.

From the Profile View

The nasion refers to the deepest point in the nasofrontal angle. The nasofrontal angle is created by the intersection of a line tangential to the infrabrow glabella and a line tangential to the pronasalae, and is measured at the nasion; it ideally ranges from 115° to 130°. The nasion labial and nasofrontal angles are shown in **Fig. 6**.

Dorsal height refers to the overall height or projection of the dorsum from the face when viewing from a profile view. Dorsal height is measured at 3 points, namely the nasion, rhinion, and tip-defining points, and they are measured in reference to the Frankfort horizontal plane (**Fig. 7**). The distance or height at the nasion is measured from the anterior corneal plane, and is ideally between 9 and 14 mm. At the rhinion it is measured from a vertical line from the alar sulcus; perpendicular to Frankfort horizontal it ideally measures between 18 and 22 mm. The ideal dorsal height at the nasal tip is between 28 and 32 mm. To simplify, one can use the 10-, 20-, 30-mm rule corresponding to nasion, rhinion, and nasal tip heights, respectively.

The radix is defined as an area whose center is at the nasion and defines the nasal root or take-off area; inferiorly it extends down to the level of a horizontal line passing through the lateral canthi. Cephalad it runs an equal distance, ideally to the level of the supratarsal crease. The ideal height

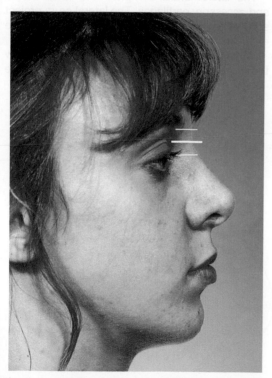

Fig. 8. Centered at the nasion, the radix extends inferiorly to the level of the lateral canthus and superiorly by an equivalent distance. (*From* Steiger JD, Baker SR. Nuances of profile management: the radix. Facial Plast Surg Clin North Am 2009;17:15–28; with permission.)

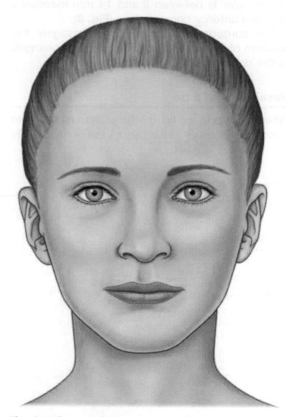

Fig. 9. When analyzing the tip, of key importance is the overall size and shape of the face, the brow-tip aesthetic line, and harmony with the alar base. (*From* Marin VP, Cochran CS, Gunter JP. Anatomic approach for tip problems. In: Aston SJ, et al, editors. Aesthetic plastic surgery. St Louis (MO): Elsevier; 2009. p. 507–21; with permission.)

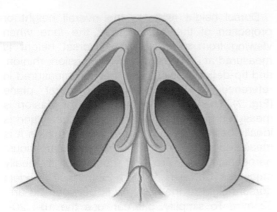

Fig. 10. The flared foot plates and the columella segment make up the components medial crura. For this reason, when analyzing the tip one must look carefully at the symmetry of the base. (*From* Daniel RK, Brenner KA. Secondary rhinoplasty. In: Aston SJ, et al, editor. Aesthetic plastic surgery. St Louis (MO): Elsevier, 2009. p. 481–94; with permission.)

of the radix is between 9 and 14 mm measured from the anterior corneal plane (**Fig. 8**).

The surgeon must thoroughly investigate the position of the radix before planning any changes to the dorsum.

Nasal Tip and Base

When analyzing the tip, the surgeon must take into account the other structures of the nose. Of key importance is the overall size and shape of the face, the brow-tip aesthetic line, and harmony with the alar base (**Fig. 9**).

When analyzing the tip one needs to document width, rotation, projection, size or volume, and definition of underlying structures.

The skin and supporting structures have to be thoroughly evaluated to determine what is surgically achievable realistically. The cartilaginous component of the nasal tip is composed of the paired alar (lower lateral) cartilages. These alar cartilages can be further divided into medial middle or intermediate and lateral crura (**Fig. 10**).

The flared foot plates and the columella segment comprise the components of the medial crura. For this reason, when analyzing the tip one must look carefully at the symmetry of the base (see **Fig. 10**). The intermediate or middle crura are composed of the lobular segment and the domal segment. Daniel further breaks down the domal segment into medial and lateral genu (see **Fig. 10**). The tip-defining points, which generally lie at the apex of the junction of the middle and lateral crus, are the most projecting points on each side of the tip; these points are responsible for the external light reflex.

The lateral crura comprise the lateral crura and accessory cartilages. The lateral crura project superolaterally to structural support to provide external nasal valve patency (**Fig. 11**).

When viewing the nasal tip from a frontal view there are 4 landmarks: the supratip break, the

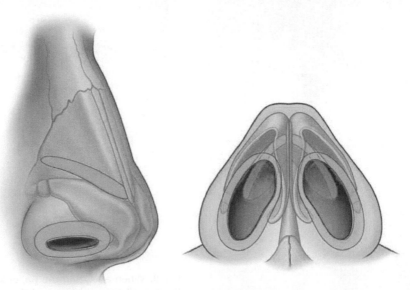

Fig. 11. The lateral crura are composed of the lateral crura and accessory cartilages. The lateral crura project superolaterally to structural support to provide external nasal valve patency. (*From* Marin VP, Cochran CS, Gunter JP. Anatomic approach for tip problems. In: Aston SJ, et al, editors. Aesthetic plastic surgery. St Louis (MO): Elsevier; 2009. p. 507–21; with permission; and Aston SJ, Martin J. Primary closed rhinoplasty. In: Aston SJ, et al, editors. Aesthetic plastic surgery. St Louis (MO): Elsevier; 2009. p. 437–72; with permission.)

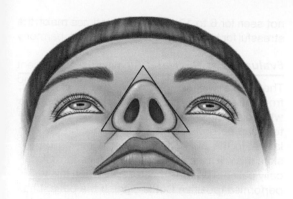

Fig. 12. The base should be in the shape of an equilateral triangle. (*From* Marin VP, Cochran CS, Gunter JP. Anatomic approach for tip problems. In: Aston SJ, et al, editors. Aesthetic plastic surgery. St Louis (MO): Elsevier; 2009. p. 507–21; with permission.)

paired tip-defining points, and the columellar lobule (see **Fig. 9**).

An aesthetic nasal tip will have a base with a width that appears to be the same as the intercanthal distance. When viewing the nose from the base, the base should create an equilateral triangle (**Fig. 12**).

Fig. 13 shows the nostril sidewall to lobular ratio. The nostrils can present in various sizes and shapes but generally are oval-triangular. The ratios of both columella and lobule to base width will affect the axis of inclination.

When drawing lines through the long axis of each nostril, they will intersect in the mid portion of the lobule Cuzalina Khan Bagheri (CKB) point. If the CKB point is caudal to the lobule it can indicate a wide base or an underprojected nose. By contrast, if the CKB point is cephalad to the lobule it can indicate a narrow base and an overprojected nose.

From a base view the ratio of the columella foot-plate complex to lobule should be 2:1 (see **Fig. 13**). The columella foot-plate complex should also be analyzed for the length of the columella and amount of lateral flaring of the foot plates. Foot plates that flare laterally from the mid columella can create a wide base and small nostrils.

The columella should curve down slightly from nasal tip to the base from a profile view, and from this view the nostril show should never be less than 1 mm or greater than 4 mm (**Fig. 14**).

The relation of the columella to the alar rim can be varied. Tip projection is the distance the nose projects from the face, and can be measured as the distance from the most posterior point of the nose-cheek junction to the tip of the nose.

Bryd described tip projection in relation to ideal nasal length (nasofrontal angle to the most anterior projecting point of the tip). When a line is drawn from the alar-cheek junction to the most anterior projecting point on the nose, this distance is 0.67 of ideal nasal length.

The Goode method of projection uses the length from the alar point to nasal tip divided by nasion to nasal tip (N-NT) length, which should ideally be 0.55 to 0.60. Crumley's method is based on

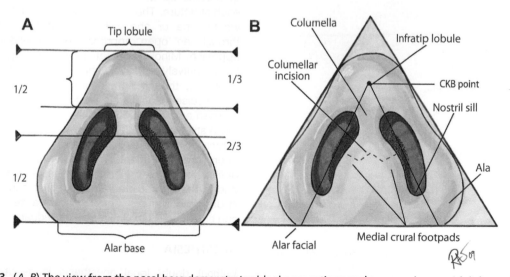

Fig. 13. (*A, B*) The view from the nasal base demonstrates ideal proportions and a general pyramidal shape that is desired. From below, the tip lobule should be approximately one-half the width of the nasal base and one-third the total projection height. The placement of a transcolumellar incision for an external rhinoplasty is made just at the top of the medial footpads. (*From* Cuzalina A. Rhinoplasty. In: Niamtu J, editor. Cosmetic facial surgery. St Louis (MO): Elsevier; 2011. p. 175–246; with permission.)

measurements that proportionately equal 3-4-5, based on lines perpendicular and parallel to the Frankfort horizontal (**Fig. 15**).

Tip grafting may improve nasal projection; however, with very thin overlying skin–soft tissue envelope the graft may become cosmetically apparent or unappealing, especially as skin undergoes age-related changes.

The surgeon must look carefully back and forth between tip and base to determine the correct surgical treatment. The most difficult task a surgeon may have is to educate a patient as to what can surgically be accomplished, as most often patients have unrealistic surgical expectations. Postsurgically the nasal tip can appear swollen, and most often the true surgical results are often

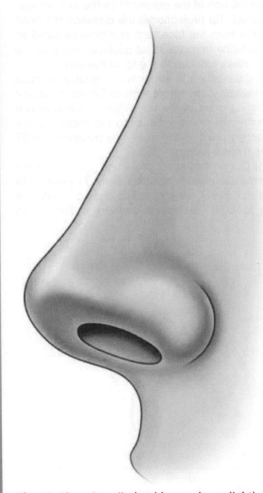

Fig. 14. The columella should curve down slightly from nasal tip to the base from a profile view, and from this view the nostril show should never be less than 1 mm or greater than 4 mm. (*From* Marin VP, Cochran CS, Gunter JP. Anatomic approach for tip problems. In: Aston SJ, et al, editors. Aesthetic plastic surgery. St Louis (MO): Elsevier; 2009. p. 507–21; with permission.)

not seen for 6 to 12 months, sometimes making it stressful for both patient and surgeon.

Evaluation of the Nasal Airway

The nasal airway can be assessed in several ways, from simply having the patient take deep breaths while pinching one nostril on either side. The Cottle test can be done by placing a finger on the skin lateral to the ala of the nose and pulling on the skin; this will assess internal valve function. Classically patients breathe much easier when this test is performed (positive Cottle sign). If the patient has internal valve compromise, the surgeon can plan for placement of spreader grafts during surgery.

Examination of the nasal speculum can help identify deflections in nasal septum as well as enlargements or asymmetries of the turbinates, bone spurs, and any inflammatory process of the nasal mucosa.

TREATMENT PLANNING

Once the patient and the surgeon have come to an agreement regarding what can surgically be achieved, the surgeon should develop a treatment plan of the surgical sequence. There are many ways through which this can be achieved; the author's preference is to list the patient's chief complaints and the patient's goals or expectations. For example, the patient may state "my nose has a big hump, it's wide and the tip points down." These complaints can then be transferred to a structural problem list, and the surgeon can then come up with a treatment plan to address each structure. The surgeon must also determine whether he or she will approach the surgery through an open approach or an endonasal approach. Minor modifications and changes can be definitively achieved through an endonasal approach, though some surgeons state that if very precise maneuvers need to be achieved then an open approach better enables these changes; this is still a topic of debate.

Ethnicity does play a major role in closed versus open surgery. Patients with darker complexions definitely tend to prefer an endonasal approach, due to the unpredictable healing that can occur in darker individuals. **Fig. 16** shows a result that can be expected in Caucasian individuals.

ANESTHESIA

Without doubt local anesthesia is needed for rhinoplasty surgery, but debate continues over whether general anesthesia or intravenous sedation should be used. Local anesthesia is required for vasoconstriction. The author has been afforded

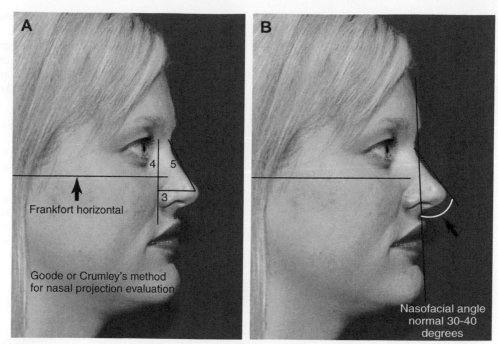

Fig. 15. (*A*) Nasal tip projection evaluation via Goode's method takes the length from alar point to nasal tip (AP-NT) divided by nasion to nasal tip (N-NT) length, which ideally should be 0.55 to 0.60. Crumley's method is based on measurement shown that should be a proportionately equal 3-4-5, based on lines perpendicular and parallel to Frankfort horizontal (3 AP-NT, 4 N line to AP, 5 N-NT). (*B*) The nasofrontal angle is glabella to nasion intersected by the N-NT line. It is likely more obtuse in females than in males. (*From* Cuzalina A. Rhinoplasty. In: Niamtu J, editor. Cosmetic facial surgery. St Louis (MO): Elsevier; 2011. p. 175–246; with permission.)

the luxury of general anesthesia during training and in practice. With the potential of blood loss to irritate the nasopharynx and oropharynx, an airway may be difficult to manage under sedation. Complex rhinoplasty requires a controlled environment especially if one needs to harvest a rib, but even so many surgeons still perform basic rhinoplasty under sedation.

In conclusion, during the initial consultation and examination the surgeon must determine whether the patient is a good candidate for rhinoplasty. Can the surgeon deliver what the patient is expecting? Ideally it is better to promise less and deliver more. The surgeon must be aware of what can be achieved with the patient's anatomy and must also understand the parameters of surgical delivery. Rhinoplasty is very challenging but, if chosen and then performed under the right circumstances, can be most rewarding and gratifying for both patient and surgeon.

SUGGESTED READINGS

Aston SJ, Martin J. Primary closed rhinoplasty. In: Aston SJ, Steinbrech DS, Walden JL, et al, editors. Aesthetic plastic surgery. St Louis (MO): Elsevier; 2009. p. 437–72.

Cuzalina A. Rhinoplasty. In: Niamtu J, editor. Cosmetic facial surgery. St Louis (MO): Elsevier; 2011. p. 175–246.

Daniel RK, Brenner KA. Secondary rhinoplasty. In: Aston SJ, Steinbrech DS, Walden JL, editors. Aesthetic plastic surgery. St Louis (MO): Elsevier; 2009. p. 481–94.

Khan HA, Bagheri SC. Initial evaluation of the cosmetic surgery patient. In: Bagher SC, Bell RB, Khan HA,

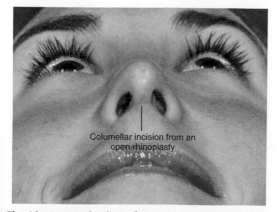

Fig. 16. Average healing of an external columellar scar 2 months following open rhinoplasty. (*From* Cuzalina A. Rhinoplasty. In: Niamtu J, editor. Cosmetic facial surgery. St Louis (MO): Elsevier; 2011. p. 175–246; with permission.)

editors. Current therapy in oral and maxillofacial surgery. Mosby (MO): Elsevier; 2011.

Koehler J. Basic rhinoplasty. In: Fonseca RJ, Turvey TA, Marciani RD, editors. Oral and maxillofacial surgery. Elsevier; 2009. p. 553–78.

Marin VP, Cochran CS, Gunter JP. Anatomic approach for tip problems. In: Aston SJ, Steinbrech DS, Walden JL, et al, editors. Aesthetic plastic surgery. St Louis (MO): Elsevier; 2009. p. 507–21.

Steiger JD, Baker SR. Nuances of profile management: the radix. Facial Plast Surg 2009;17(1):15–28.

Toriumi DM, Checcone MA. New concepts in nasal tip contouring. Facial Plast Surg 2009;17(1): 55–90.

Applied Surgical Anatomy of the Nose

Mark R. Stevens, DDS*, Hany A. Emam, BDS, MS

KEYWORDS

- Anatomy • Nose • Surgery • Lower lateral cartilage
- Upper lateral cartilage • Nasal septum

Although anatomy often seems static, the continual innovation of new surgical techniques and approaches, in reality, make it a dynamic field. The first essential principal of any surgery is the comprehensive knowledge of the anatomic area and its physiology. This assertion is especially true in functional and or cosmetic nasal surgery.

The list of adjectives to describe the nose are limitless; "ballooned," "defined," "gallant," "alluring," "eagle-like," "button," and "turned up" are just a few. This short list emphasizes the varied anatomic forms and why the nose is such an important component of facial appearance, even implying one's personality. Manipulation of the nose is a challenging endeavor because of the varied forms. The surgeon must not only comprehend the three-dimensional structural aspects of the nose but also understand the properties and behavior of different tissue types to achieve long-term predictable results. A thorough understanding of applied surgical anatomy allows for optimum access, visualization, cosmetics, and functionality during surgical manipulations.

EXTERNAL NOSE

The nose is a complex structure that can be subdivided topographically into thirds and functional cosmetic units. The anatomic thirds of the nose are best viewed from several vantage points. The frontal, lateral, and basal views are all required to adequately assess the nasal structures (**Figs. 1–3**). The upper one-third, or nasion region, contains the paired nasal bones. The nasal bones vary greatly in length. They are approximately 2.5 cm long and become thinner as they extend caudally toward the rhinion.[1,2] The nasal bones are attached to the frontal bone superiorly, which corresponds topographically to the radix or root of the nose. The radix forms an obtuse angle with the frontal bone, which varies with gender. The nasal bones articulate with the lacrimal bones superolaterally, and the nasomaxillary processes inferolaterally. Nasal bones overlap the upper lateral cartilages caudally. This special relationship is discussed in more detail. The intercanthal tendon splits the dorsal length of the nasal bones approximately in half.[3,4] This anatomic structure is important when performing lateral nasal osteotomy during rhinoplasty procedures.

The middle one-third of the nose contains the paired upper lateral cartilages (ULCs), also referred to as the *cartilaginous vault region*. The ULCs are fused superiorly but separate from the septum as they extend inferiorly.[5] Laterally they become more rectangular in shape. The ULCs do not rest on the piriform process, as was earlier thought, but rather end in a region called the *external lateral triangle of the piriform aperture*.[6] This area also contains small sesamoid cartilages and may aid in respiration as a bellows (see **Figs. 1** and **2**).[7]

The lower one-third or lobule can be further subdivided into three parts topographically: the tip and the supra and infra tips. These specific areas of the lobule are formed from the varied shape, size, and angles of the lower lateral cartilages (LLCs). The LLCs are presently divided into three distinct regions: medial, middle, and lateral, and are discussed later in more detail. From a lateral

Oral and Maxillofacial Surgery Department, Georgia Health Sciences University College of Dental Medicine, 1430 John Wesley Gilbert Drive, Room GC1055A, Augusta, GA 30912, USA
* Corresponding author.
E-mail address: mastevens@georgiahealth.edu

Oral Maxillofacial Surg Clin N Am 24 (2012) 25–38
doi:10.1016/j.coms.2011.10.007
1042-3699/12/$ – see front matter © 2012 Elsevier Inc. All rights reserved.

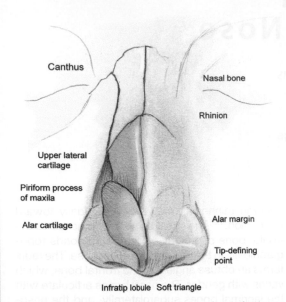

Fig. 1. Frontal view of the bony and cartilaginous nasal structures.

view, the lobule is defined by the tip or apex of the nose. The cephalic edge of the domal segment of the middle crus is responsible for the esthetic point known as the *pronasale*. The supra tip is immediately cephalic to the pronasale. The infra tip is located between the pronasale and the base of the nostrils. The lower one-third of the nose has various thicknesses of fibro fatty connective tissue. The thickness of this soft tissue envelope often masks the defined lobular features. The infra tip region should have a gentle curve that slightly projects inferiorly to the alar margins (see **Figs. 1** and **2**).[3,8]

The basal view gives an important perspective when accessing the medial and middle crura of the LLCs. Deformities of the caudal septum may also be observed from this view (see **Fig. 3**).

Esthetically acceptable anthropometric measurements from different views provided useful information in planning rhinoplasty procedures. Frontally, the length of the nose to that of the middle third of the face is 90%. The ratio of the nasal root width to the alar width is 50%. The nasal projection on profile is 40% of the nasal length,

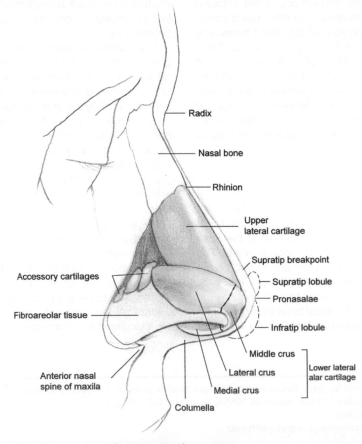

Fig. 2. Lateral view of the bony and cartilaginous nasal structures.

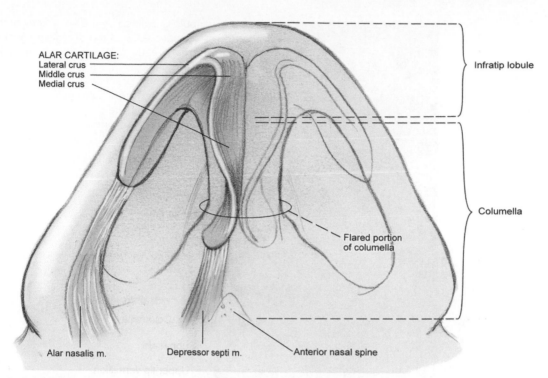

ALAR CARTILAGE:
Lateral crus
Middle crus
Medial crus

Infratip lobule

Columella

Flared portion
of columella

Alar nasalis m.

Depressor septi m.

Anterior nasal spine

Fig. 3. Basal view of the bony and cartilaginous nasal structures. m, muscle.

and the nasal tip length is 45% of nasal projection. The nasal projection is also 60% of both alar width and alar length (**Fig. 4**).[9]

SOFT TISSUE ENVELOPE

The nose is composed of a wide composite of tissues types, including skin, dermis, muscular fascia, fibro fatty, mucosa, cartilage, perichondrium, bone and periosteum. The overlying soft tissue varies greatly in its thicknesses, attachments, and compositions, especially among different ethnicities.[10] This differential helped define the nasal subunits first described by Gonzalez-Ulloa and colleagues[2] (**Fig. 5**). The skin thickness average is 1.25 mm at the nasofrontal area or radix and the thinnest at the rhinion at 0.6 mm.[1]

The soft tissue mobility also plays an important role in the dynamics of the anatomy, function, facial expressions, and subsequent manipulations of the nose. The skin, dermis, and subcutaneous tissue move freely over the upper two-thirds of the nose because of extension of the superficial musculoaponeurotic system (SMAS).[11] The skin and fatty tissue, however, attaches firmly over the lower one-third of the nose, including the tip. The skin in this area also contains a great amount of exocrine glands, such as sebaceous

and sweat glands. The importance of assessing the tips' soft tissue volume and consistency cannot be overemphasized for achieving the desired esthetic results in rhinoplasty. Unless one is debulking excessive fibrofatty tissue from the nose, the optimum avascular plane of dissection is in the supraperichondreal plane just below the fibrofatty SMAS layer.[12]

The lining of the nose transforms from stratified squamous keratinized epithelium at the nasal vestibule to a psuedostratified columnar ciliated epithelium as the surgeon regresses internally. The overlying mucosa of the anterior septum and the inferior turbinate contain specially adapted erectile tissue composed of multiple venous sinusoids that can be quickly filled and drained to permit rapid variations in the cross-sectional area of the nasal valve regulating air flow and moisture exchange.[13] Atraumatic dissection of the nasal mucosa should be performed to prevent perforation and scaring.

MUSCULATURE

The muscles of animation of the nose are divided by their functions into four categories: elevators, depressors, compressors, and dilators.[14] The procerus, levator labii superioris alaeque nasi, and anomalous nasi elevate and shorten the nose.

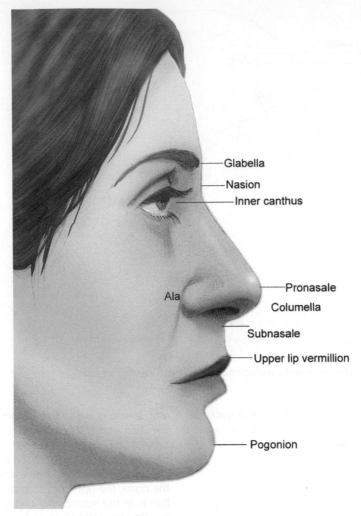

Glabella

Nasion

Inner canthus

Pronasale

Ala

Columella

Subnasale

Upper lip vermillion

Pogonion

Fig. 4. Soft tissue landmarks for the nose. Profile view.

These muscles are important because they assist in the opening of the nasal valves. The depressor muscles consist of the nasalis and depressor septi. On animation, this group of muscles adversely affects tip projection by displacing it inferiorly and elevating the lip superiorly **(Fig. 6)**.[15]

SENSORY NERVE SUPPLY

The external nose receives its sensation from two divisions of the trigeminal nerve: the ophthalmic (V1) and maxillary (V2) nerve distributions. The external nose sensory dermatomes have been described as an island of V1 in a sea of V2. The ophthalmic division has three main branches: the lacrimal, frontal, and nasocilliary. The lacrimal and nasocilliary innervate the lateral and medial orbit.

The frontal nerve further divides into the supraorbital and supratrochlear. These nerves provide sensation to the forehead and nasion region, respectively. The nasocilliary nerve is definitively smaller than the other two branches. Its terminal branch becomes the external nasal nerve. The external nasal branch, before exiting between the lower border of the nasal bone and the lateral nasal cartilage, is the anterior ethmoidal nerve responsible for sensation of the anterior superior aspect of the internal nose. The external nasal nerve supplies the skin of the dorsum, ala, and apex of the nose.[5] Injury to this nerve occurs when dissection is deep to the supraperichondreal plane, resulting in persistent numbness to the lateral ala and tip of the nose **(Fig. 7)**.[1,5]

The maxillary division (V2) is divided into six branches: maxillary, sphenopalatine, zygomatic, superior posterior alveolar, superior anterior

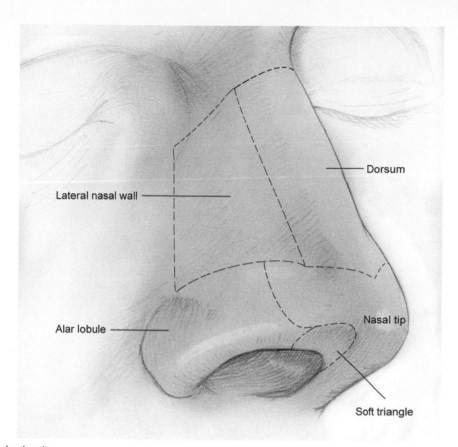

Fig. 5. Nasal subunits.

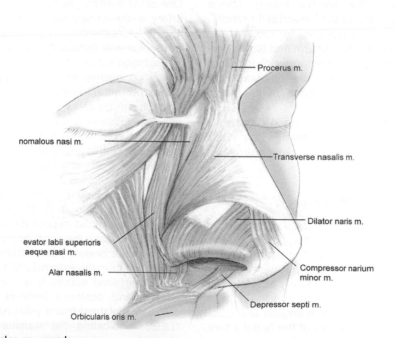

Fig. 6. Nasal muscles. m, muscle.

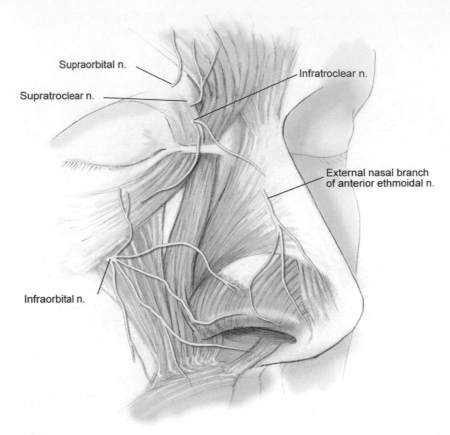

Fig. 7. Nerves of the nose. n, nerve.

alveolar (mediates the sneeze reflex), lateral external nares, and finally the infraorbital branch.

The maxillary branch provides for most of the sensation along the lateral dorsum and ala bilaterally. The sphenopalatine nerve further divides into lateral and septal branches. It gives sensation to the posterior and central regions of the nasal cavity.

Other cranially nerves of importance in the nose are the facial (VII), which innervates the nasal musculature, and the olfactory (I), which provides the sense of smell.[1,5]

BLOOD SUPPLY TO THE NOSE

The nose, like the rest of the face, has significant vascular redundancy. The blood supply originates from the internal and external carotid arteries. The major blood supply to the external nose is from three vessels: the dorsal nasal artery as a terminal branch of the ophthalmic artery, and the angular and superior labial arteries. The angular and labial arteries are terminal branches of the facial artery, which originates off the external carotid artery.

One of the terminal branches of the superior labial artery is the columellar branch. This branch is always encountered and transected during open transcolumellar rhinoplasty approaches.[5,16,17]

The blood supply of the internal nasal cavity has numerous overlapping intertwining connections. The upper septal blood supply comes from the anterior and posterior ethmoidal arteries and the sphenopalatine artery. Anteriorly, the septum and nasal floor is vascularized by terminal branches of the superior labial artery. The lateral nasal cavities are similarly highly vascularized. The blood supply can also be divided into posterior and anterior regions. Posteriorly, the blood supply arises from the maxillary artery and its terminal branches. Laterally, the blood supply comes from multiple sources, including the superior nasal, greater palatine, superior alveolar, and infraorbital arteries, all originating from the external carotid artery.[18] Anteriorly, the blood supply is a combination of the anterior and posterior terminal branches. This confluence of these four arteries has the mnemonic "LEGS," indicating the superior labial, anterior ethmoidal, greater palatine, and sphenopalatine arteries. This confluence of arteries anteriorly along the septum is called *Kesselbach's plexus*, and is an area prone to chronic anterior nose bleeds (**Fig. 8**).[6,18]

The venous drainage of the nose basically follows the arterial supply. Venous drainage occurs through three major regions: the pharyngeal and pterygoid plexus posteriorly, and the facial vein anteriorly. The significant anatomic feature of these veins is their lack of internal valves and their potential to carry infection backward toward the cavernous sinus and brain.

LYMPHATIC DRAINAGE

The anterior nasal lymphatics drain anteriorly to the upper lip lymphatics. Posteriorly, drainage passes toward the deep cervical and retropharyngeal lymph nodes.[5]

INTERNAL NOSE

The nasal cavity is a unique and highly specialized structural organ. The nose provides for humidification and warming of inspired air, filtration, smell, and resonation of sounds.[19]

NASAL SEPTUM

The nasal septum is a composite structure in the midline made of a flat cartilaginous part anteriorly and a bony part posteriorly. The anterior part is an irregular quadrangular made of hyaline cartilage. The posterior bony part is composed of four bones: the vomer, the perpendicular plate of

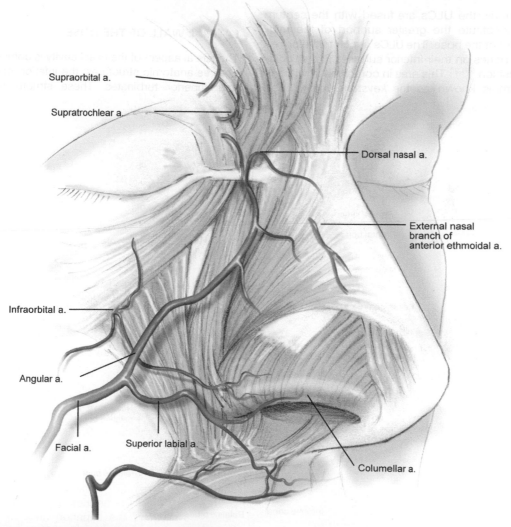

Supraorbital a.

Supratrochlear a.

Dorsal nasal a.

External nasal branch of anterior ethmoidal a.

Infraorbital a.

Angular a.

Facial a.

Superior labial a.

Columellar a.

Fig. 8. Arterial blood supply to the nose. a, artery.

the ethmoid bone, and the maxillary and palatine bones (**Fig. 9**).[5]

The quadrangular cartilaginous septum varies greatly in sizes and is prone to deformation. It is responsible for the support and form of the nasal dorsum from it junction at rhinion to the lobule at the supratip break. Internally and inferiorly the quadrangular septum is attached tightly and insets into the nasomaxillary crest of the maxilla and nasal spine.[5,20] This fusion of both the periosteum and perichondrium often make dissection difficult in sepal surgery, especially when the septum has been deviated to one side.[8] When performing cartilaginous septal manipulation with resection, a 1-cm segment of caudal and dorsal cartilage should be maintained to provide internal nasal support.

ULC

Superiorly, the ULCs are fused with the septum and constitute the greater support of the mid-dorsum of the nose. The ULCs attach to the paired nasal bones on their inferior surfaces in a shingle-like fashion.[5,6,21] This area in combination with the septum is known as the *keystone region*. The amount of overlap varies, but it can be as great as 1 cm in length.[22–24] The importance of maintaining this relationship cannot be overstated in rhinoplasty.

The ULCs also play an essential role in the makeup of the internal nasal valve. Careful dissection of the mucosa (extramucosal) from the ULCs is critical to prevent adhesions, synechiae, and thus narrowing of the internal nasal valve.[25] The caudal area of the ULC and its relationship with the LLCs is also referred to as the *scroll region*.[25] The ULCs and LLCs at the scroll area have a fibrous attachment. This attachment has been mentioned as one of the minor support mechanisms of the nasal tip. Several anatomic variations have been illustrated describing this unique connection.[6,14,15] The degree of the slope of the lateral crus cephalic edge and size of the scroll area determines the bulbous nature of the lobule (**Fig. 10**).[6]

LATERAL WALL OF THE NOSE

The lateral aspect of the nasal cavity is composed of three anatomic structures: the inferior, middle, and superior turbinates. These structures are

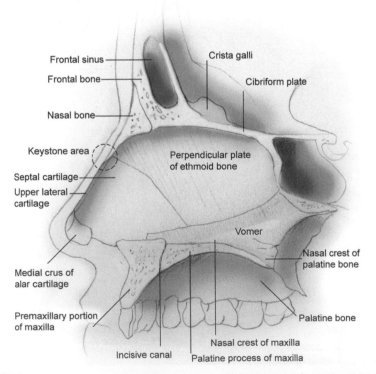

Fig. 9. Nasal septum.

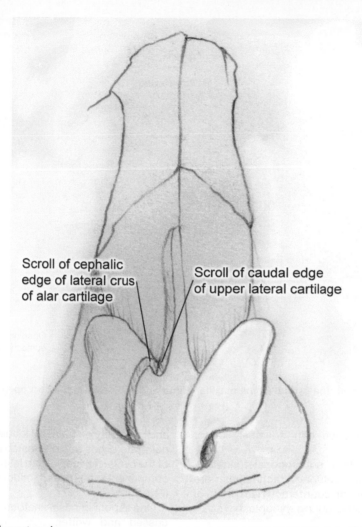

Scroll of cephalic edge of lateral crus of alar cartilage

Scroll of caudal edge of upper lateral cartilage

Fig. 10. Scroll attachment region.

important for filtering, humidifying, and warming inspired air. The inferior turbinate is a single bone, whereas the middle and upper turbinates are extensions of the ethmoid bone.[1] The inferior turbinate impinges on the internal nasal valve region, where its specially adapted erectile tissues regulate the air flow and facilitate heat and moisture exchange. Although air flow dynamics is critical for normal nasal physiology and functioning, controversy remains regarding the precise nature of the normal nasal air pattern flow. The inferior turbinate seem to participate in the generation of a turbulent air flow that seems to be more physiologic than laminar air flow.[13] Turbinates, especially the inferior one, often require concomitant surgery during rhinoplasty, particularly in reduction rhinoplasty procedures.[26] These structures also have associated meatus for sinus and lacrimal drainages. Careful surgical manipulation is required to ensure no damage or blockage of these openings **(Fig. 11)**.[20]

INTERNAL NASAL VALVE

The internal nasal valve is anatomically defined as an angle located at the junction between the ULCs and the LLCs and their relationship with the septum.[18,19] This angle varies between 10° and 15°. Its shape and size depend on an individual's ethnicity **(Fig. 12)**.[26]

Small changes or decreases in its shape can severely affect internal nasal air flow. Described by Poiseuille's law, the valve area is proportional to the radius raised to the fourth power. Therefore, small changes to the valve's cross-sectional area can exponentially increase airflow resistance.[25] The LLCs often overlap to some extent, which helps support the internal valve function.

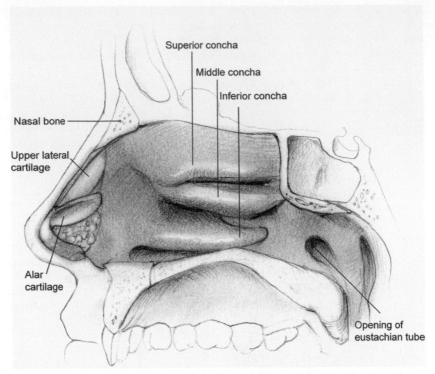

Fig. 11. Lateral nasal wall. The ostium of the maxillary sinus and the nasolacrimal duct opening are obscured by the turbinates.

Therefore, LLC reduction can adversely affect valve function.

Atraumatic dissection, submucosal tunneling, grafting, or unique suturing techniques are required to maintain or counteract narrowing of the internal nasal valves during rhinoplasty.[25]

LLCS AND THE TIP OF THE NOSE

The LLCs are divided into distinct regions because of their importance in providing the unique shape and variability of the nasal lobule. Many expert rhinologists divide the long-established two portions of the LLC—the medial and lateral crus—into three components: the lateral, middle, and medial crus **(Fig. 13).**[23,27]

One aspect of nasal anatomy that has been discussed and written about excessively is the anatomy and surgical manipulation of the nasal

Fig. 12. Anatomy of the internal nasal valve.

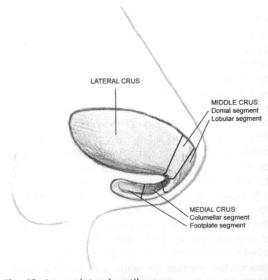

Fig. 13. Lower lateral cartilages.

tip structures. Anatomically, the lower third of the nose consists of the lobule, columella, nostril floors, vestibules, alar bases, and side walls. The three major tip components are the crural complexes (LLCs) themselves, with the structure defined by their size, shape, position, and ligamentous and fibrous attachments.[28]

Medial Crus

The medial crus consists of the columellar and footplate segments. These segments are responsible for the angulation, divergence, and shape of the nasal base. Well-projected noses result from an elongation of the columella segment of the medial crus. Several constant variations exist in the columella segment, according to cadaveric studies by Dingman and Natvig.[29] The nasal base anatomy and shape are dependent on not only these variations but also the interaction with the caudal nasal septum, varied soft tissue thickness, and footplate component.

Middle (Intermediate) Crus

The middle region of the LLC is referred to as the intermediate crus. The middle and medial crura are attached to each other by a fibrous transverse thickening known as the interdomal ligament. The middle crus is further subdivided anatomically and cosmetically into a domal and a lobular segment.[8] The lobular portion's length, shape, and angulations are responsible for the infratip lobule's form. The domal portion of the intermediate crus also varies greatly in shape. It is usually short and often the most delicate portion of the LLCs. Its inherent weakness in this region can be responsible for notching of the soft tissue triangle.[28,30]

The domal portion of the intermediate crus defines points of the nasal tip. These points are a result of the cephalic edges of the cartilages as they diverge and slope posteriorly.[30]

Both regions may require augmentation to achieve this defined pattern, especially after refining manipulations (**Fig. 14**).

The domal portions of the middle crus are tightly bound together by the interdomal ligament. Pitanguy[31] also describes a vertical orientation of fibers in this area to the overlying soft tissue called the dermocartilaginous ligament. These ligamentous structures are minor mechanisms in elevating and maintaining support of the lobule (**Fig. 15**).

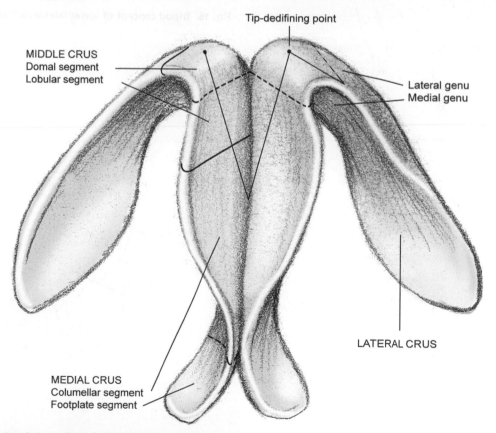

Tip-dedifining point

MIDDLE CRUS
Domal segment
Lobular segment

Lateral genu
Medial genu

LATERAL CRUS

MEDIAL CRUS
Columellar segment
Footplate segment

Fig. 14. Basal view of medial and middle crura.

Lateral Crus

The lateral crus is the largest and strongest component of the LLCs, and thus plays the major role in supporting the lobule. The size and contour of the lower lateral cartilages vary greatly among ethnicities. Non-Caucasians, often referred to as having a platyrrhine nose, have a shorter and weaker medial and lateral crus compared with the larger lateral crus seen in an aquiline, or beaked-type, noses. The LLCs also provide an important element in the shape of the alar side wall. The shape of the lateral crus plays an important aspect in the cosmetic outcome. On cadaveric review, Zelnik and Gingrass[32] described specific contours in the convexity or concavity of the lateral crus and their relationship to creating an esthetic lobule. They concluded that convexity

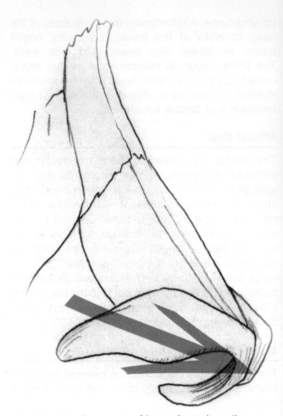

Fig. 16. Tripod concept of lower lateral cartilages.

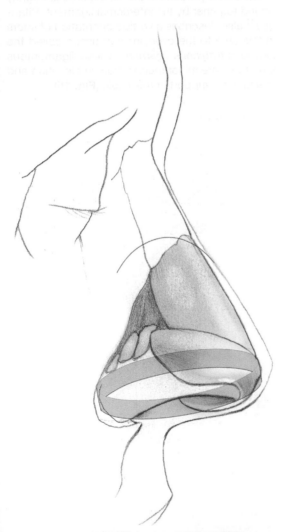

Fig. 15. Dermocartilaginous ring of the lobule.

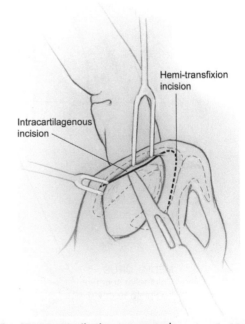

Hemi-transfixion incision

Intracartilagenous incision

Fig. 17. Intracartilaginous approach.

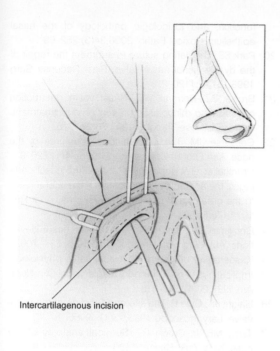

Intercartilagenous incision

Fig. 18. Intercartilaginous approach.

of the lateral crus is associated with a more favorable outcome when creating an acute and defined domal angle. Hafezi and colleagues[33] described a three-dimensional hemispheric form to the LLC, with an inward limb attaching to the ULC at the scroll area in 40% of noses undergoing open rhinoplasty. This anatomic variant is responsible for asymmetry and flaring of the nostril.

The shape and stiffness of the lateral crus in combination with the fibrous support mechanism of the lower nose are considered to be responsible for the primary internal support of the tip. The lower alar cartilages, in combination with the other suspensory complexes (eg, domal and septal ligaments) and in association with fibrous attachment at the piriform, form a ring-like structure. These alar cartilages are responsible for the overall characteristics of the nasal apertures.[34]

The LLCs and their combined support contribute to the concept of a tripod-like structure. The fibrous connection between the middle and medial crura are considered one leg of the tripod, with the lateral crura forming the other two legs.[35] This tripod theory was first espoused by Anderson[36] in the 1960s, and still plays a dynamic role in the cantilevering of the nasal tip in cosmetic rhinoplasty (**Fig. 16**).

SURGICAL APPROACHES

A multitude of surgical approaches are available for accessing the nose, depending on the area of manipulation and severity of nasal deformities and associated structures. Most cosmetic approaches are through the lower two-thirds of the nose. These approaches can be grouped as endonasal or external. The major approaches for rhinoplasty include transcolumellar, transfixion, hemitransfixion, infracartilaginous (marginal), intercartilaginous, and cartilage-splitting incisions.[6,37–39] The transcolumellar approach is becoming more common because it allows increased visualization and avoids internal nasal scaring from combined multiple endonasal incisions.[40]

The multiple approaches in rhinoplasty usually depend on the surgeon's experience and training, and the complexity of the deformity. Complex cases involving multiple structures, such as septum, skeleton, and tip, require open techniques.

Figs. 17–19 depict the most common rhinoplasty approaches to the nasal skeleton.

ACKNOWLEDGMENTS

The authors want to express their sincere gratitude to Begonia Rueda Rodriquez for her accurate anatomical depictions. They truly add to the article's value by highlighting the important anatomical

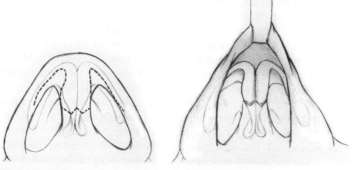

Fig. 19. Transcolumellar open approach.

structures as they relate to the applied surgical anatomy of the nose.

REFERENCES

1. Oneal RM, Beil RJ. Surgical anatomy of the nose. Clin Plast Surg 2010;37(2):191–211.
2. Gonzalez-Ulloa M, Castillo A, Stevens E, et al. Preliminary study of the total restoration of the facial skin. Plast Reconstr Surg (1946) 1954;13(3):151–61.
3. Lessard ML, Daniel RK. Surgical anatomy of septo-rhinoplasty. Arch Otolaryngol 1985;111(1):25–9.
4. Wright WK. Surgery of the bony and cartilaginous dorsum. Otolaryngol Clin North Am 1975;8(3):575–98.
5. Hollingshead WH, editor. 3rd edition, Anatomy for surgeons, vol. 1. Philadelphia: Harper and Row; 1982.
6. Johnson CM, Toriumi DM. Open structure rhinoplasty. Philadelphia: WB Saunders; 1990.
7. Bernstein L. Surgical anatomy in rhinoplasty. Otolaryngol Clin North Am 1975;8(3):549–58.
8. Schlosser RJ, Park SS. Functional nasal surgery. Otolaryngol Clin North Am 1999;32(1):37–51.
9. Epker BN. Evaluation of the face. In: Fonseca RJ, Marciani RD, Turvey TA, editors. Oral and maxillofacial surgery. 2nd edition. St Louis (MO): Saunders-Elsevier; 2009. p. 1–59.
10. Peck GC, Michelson LN. Anatomy of aesthetic surgery of the nose. Clin Plast Surg 1987;14(4):737–48.
11. Letourneau A, Daniel RK. The superficial musculoaponeurotic system of the nose. Plast Reconstr Surg 1988;82(1):48–57.
12. Gunter RA, Rohisch RJ, Adams WP. Dallas rhinoplasty: nasal surgery by the masters. 2nd edition. St Louis (MO): Quality Medical publishing; 2007.
13. Snow JB, Wackym PA. Ballenger's otorhinolaryngology head and neck surgery. 17th edition. Shelton (CT): People's Medical Publishing House; 2009.
14. Gruber RP, Freeman MB, Hsu C, et al. Nasal base reduction by alar release: a laboratory evaluation. Plast Reconstr Surg 2009;123(2):709–15.
15. Clark MP, Greenfield B, Hunt N, et al. Function of the nasal muscles in normal subjects assessed by dynamic MRI and EMG: its relevance to rhinoplasty surgery. Plast Reconstr Surg 1998;101(7):1945–55.
16. Herbert DC. A subcutaneous pedicled cheek flap for reconstruction of alar defects. Br J Plast Surg 1978;31(2):79–92.
17. Rohrich RJ, Gunter JP, Friedman RM. Nasal tip blood supply: an anatomic study validating the safety of the transcolumellar incision in rhinoplasty. Plast Reconstr Surg 1995;95(5):795–9 [discussion: 800–1].
18. Oneal RM, Beil RJ Jr, Schlesinger J. Surgical anatomy of the nose. Otolaryngol Clin North Am 1999;32(1):145–81.
19. Harkema JR, Carey SA, Wagner JG. The nose revisited: a brief review of the comparative structure, function, and toxicologic pathology of the nasal epithelium. Toxicol Pathol 2006;34(3):252–69.
20. Park SS. The flaring suture to augment the repair of the dysfunctional nasal valve. Plast Reconstr Surg 1998;101(4):1120–2.
21. Broker BJ, Berman WE. Nasal valve obstruction complicating rhinoplasty: prevention and treatment. Part I. Ear Nose Throat J 1997;76(2):77–8.
22. Converse JM. The cartilaginous structures of the nose. Ann Otol Rhinol Laryngol 1955;64(1):220–9.
23. Drumheller GW. Topology of the lateral nasal cartilages: the anatomical relationship of the lateral nasal to the greater alar cartilage, lateral crus. Anat Rec 1973;176(3):321–7.
24. Converse JM. Corrective surgery of nasal deviations. AMA Arch Otolaryngol 1950;52(5):671–708.
25. Kasperbauer JL, Kern EB. Nasal valve physiology. Implications in nasal surgery. Otolaryngol Clin North Am 1987;20(4):699–719.
26. Haight JS, Cole P. The site and function of the nasal valve. Laryngoscope 1983;93(1):49–55.
27. Tardy ME Jr, Brown RJ. Surgical anatomy of the nose. New York: Raven; 1990.
28. Daniel RK. The nasal tip: anatomy and aesthetics. Plast Reconstr Surg 1992;89(2):216–24.
29. Dingman RO, Natvig P. Surgical anatomy in aesthetic and corrective rhinoplasty. Clin Plast Surg 1977;4(1):111–20.
30. Tardy ME Jr, Patt BS, Walter MA. Transdomal suture refinement of the nasal tip: long-term outcomes. Facial Plast Surg 1993;9(4):275–84.
31. Pitanguy I. Surgical importance of a dermocartilaginous ligament in bulbous noses. Plast Reconstr Surg 1965;36:247–53.
32. Zelnik J, Gingrass RP. Anatomy of the alar cartilage. Plast Reconstr Surg 1979;64(5):650–3.
33. Hafezi F, Naghibzadeh B, Nouhi AH. Applied anatomy of the nasal lower lateral cartilage: a new finding. Aesthetic Plast Surg 2010;34(2):244–8.
34. Farkas LG, Hreczko TA, Deutsch CK. Objective assessment of standard nostril types—a morphometric study. Ann Plast Surg 1983;11(5):381–9.
35. Burget GC, Menick FJ. Nasal support and lining: the marriage of beauty and blood supply. Plast Reconstr Surg 1989;84(2):189–202.
36. Anderson JR. New approach to rhinoplasty. A five-year reappraisal. Arch Otolaryngol 1971;93(3):284–91.
37. Sheen JH, Sheen AP. Aesthetic rhinoplasty. 2nd edition. St Louis (MO): Mosby; 1987.
38. Daniel RK. Aesthetic plastic surgery-rhinoplasty. Boston: Little, Brown & Co; 1993.
39. Guida RA. Surgical approaches to the nasal skeleton. Operat Tech Otolaryngol Head Neck Surg 1999;10:228–31.
40. Waite PD. Avoiding revision rhinoplasty. Oral Maxillofac Surg Clin North Am 2011;23(1):93–100, vi.

Primary Cosmetic Rhinoplasty

Shahrokh C. Bagheri, DMD, MD

KEYWORDS

- Rhinoplasty • Cosmetic • Nasal structure
- Nose modification

The last 2 decades have witnessed significant contributions to rhinoplasty, which have changed both technical and philosophic aspects of rhinoplasty surgery. Many of these changes are designed to provide more predictable, lasting, and enhanced cosmetic results of surgery without compromise of function. In comparison with many branches of surgery rhinoplasty remains in its infancy, and because of the lack of evidence-based advancement of this discipline using randomized studies, the field continues to evolve through the experience and sharing of surgical knowledge of individual surgeons, educational symposiums, hands-on courses, textbooks, and peer-reviewed publications that predominantly include case reports, case series, and technical notes. Although the aim of this procedure remains unchanged, the techniques and methodology have evolved. What is also continuously changing is patients' requests and expectations of favorable cosmetic outcomes. This article outlines the basic concepts that are essential in performing cosmetic rhinoplasty.

Primary cosmetic rhinoplasty refers to the surgical manipulation of the previously unoperated nose for esthetic enhancement. A history of septoplasty in the absence of any cosmetic nasal alterations may change the treatment plan related to septal harvest, yet the procedure remains a primary cosmetic rhinoplasty, distinguished from revision and reconstructive rhinoplasty. In a revision procedure, the surgeon attempts to correct or further modify a previously operated nose. A revision procedure can be indicated if the patient and clinician agree that the expected or planned results were not obtained from the primary procedure, or if results are compromised

because of complications. This procedure is further distinguished from a repeat or redo rhinoplasty whereby a patient presents after a primary rhinoplasty requesting changes from a previously satisfactory result. Reconstructive rhinoplasty is the esthetic and/or functional enhancement of a nose that is altered by trauma, pathology, or ablative tumor surgery.

The difficulty of rhinoplasty is attributed to the complex anatomy of the area involving cartilage, bony structures, and a skin-soft tissue envelope (S-STE) (**Fig. 1**). **Table 1** summarizes the anatomic regions of the nose and their main characteristics for cosmetic and functional rhinoplasty. The central position of the nose and its intimate relationships with peripheral facial features such as the extension of the dorsum with the brow lines, malar projection, columellar support, or esthetic projection of the chin on profile are important esthetic features that contribute to facial beauty. The alteration of the nose cannot be planned solely in conjunction with the nasal anatomy (radix, septum, dorsum, tip, base) but in relation to the rest of the face. This notion is further challenged by a relatively small margin of error for optimal results and the integration of successful functional outcomes in view of the cosmetic result, which frequently involves the desire for a smaller nose while maintaining nasal airway patency. Furthermore, unlike with most facial cosmetic procedures, the patients presenting for primary cosmetic rhinoplasty are frequently young adults. Younger patients' desire for rhinoplasty may not be as clearly communicated or foreseen, and in the authors' opinion can be readily confounded by the opinion and influence of parents, friends, and current social and ethnic norms; this can result

Georgia Oral and Facial Surgery, and Eastern Surgical Associates and Consultants, 1880 West Oak Parkway, Suite 215, Marietta, GA 30062, USA
E-mail address: sbagher@hotmail.com

Oral Maxillofacial Surg Clin N Am 24 (2012) 39–48
doi:10.1016/j.coms.2011.10.001

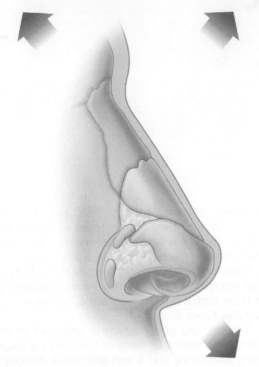

Fig. 1. Anatomy of nasal structures as seen from profile. (*From* Bagheri SC, Jo C. Clinical review of oral and maxillofacial surgery. Mosby/Elsevier; 2008. p. 308; with permission.)

in the development of unclear and unrealistic expectations. In addition, a rhinoplasty may be the patient's first experience of cosmetic surgery, therefore contributing to the difficulty in the management of anxiety, expectations, pain management, and overall experience.

Table 1
Anatomic regions of the nose and their main characteristics for cosmetic and functional rhinoplasty

Anatomic Region	Main Characteristics
Radix	Location, size
Dorsum	Width, size, symmetry
Tip	Volume, projection, shape, definition, rotation, width
Nasal base	Alar base shape, nostril size, columellar anatomy, alar width, symmetry
Septum	Deviation, perforation
Turbinates	Size, obstruction of airflow, inflammation

Data from Bagheri SC, Khan HA. Current trends in rhinoplasty. In: Bagheri SC, Bell RB, Khan HA, editors. Current therapy in Oral and maxillofacial surgery. St Louis (MO): Saunders; 2012.

Ultimately a successful cosmetic rhinoplasty requires that the patient clearly communicates the desire and expectations for surgery. The surgeon must take the time to understand and recognize unrealistic requests, ambiguity, and contradictions in the patient's desire. Subsequently, the surgeon must have a complete grasp of the surgical maneuvers at his or her disposal and be able to translate them into a custom operation that meets the patient's requests. It is essential that the surgeon recognize that each surgical intervention has a standard range of applications and error margin that can cause deviations from the planned procedure. The more complex is the set of interventions, the greater the margin of error. The current principles of rhinoplasty emphasize the adherence to minor but key changes that result in more predictable and lasting outcomes. When possible, surgeons should evaluate their results beyond the first 6 to 12 months, although to a lesser extent the nose will continue to change beyond this period. The stability of the cosmetic result will depend on the degree of cartilaginous, ligamentous, bony, and soft-tissue disruption, and surgically designed structural modifications. Long-term results can be difficult to decipher not only because of difficulty in follow-up but also because the nose continues to age along with the other facial structures.

THE EVOLUTION OF RHINOPLASTY TECHNIQUES

Rhinoplasty has evolved based on advancements in surgical technique that have survived the test of time and increasing patient expectations. Cosmetic surgery is unique among other surgical specialties because of changing trends, and racial and regional ethnic preferences that drive the patient's desires toward what is considered an esthetic result. In no other procedure are such differences so evident as for rhinoplasty. The operation is individually customized to account for current ethnic and cultural norms. In modern rhinoplasty surgery, no single procedure or approach can provide such a vast array of patient desires for beauty and functionality. Surgeons have to be armed with multiple techniques based on patient demands that are used in concert to give predictable results. Cosmetic rhinoplasty remains one of the most challenging facial cosmetic procedures, and this is unlikely to change despite many advances and alterations in the field.

Many of the fundamental principles of cosmetic rhinoplasty have evolved since the popularization of this procedure in the last 40 years. Initially rhinoplasty was primarily performed as a reductive procedure, focused on removal of the dorsum and cartilage excision. More recently, cartilage grafting and advanced suturing techniques have caused a paradigm shift toward tissue preservation and anatomic form. The concept of balanced rhinoplasty refers to alterations of nasal anatomy by reduction, augmentation, or alteration to achieve the anatomic harmony between the radix, dorsum, tip, and alar base. The surgical access to the nasal structures has also seen the dramatic popularization of the open approach.

Patients who seek cosmetic rhinoplasty are often confused by the variety of surgical disciplines that offer this procedure. The capability to perform rhinoplasty is no longer dictated by specialty but by surgical training.

The desire to perform rhinoplasty is generally dictated by several factors. Congenitally or acquired (via trauma) nasal deformities such as crooked, deviated, or collapsed nasal structures are common etiological factors in cosmetic rhinoplasty. Such deformities are frequently combined with functional disturbances (most commonly deviated septum causing impaired air flow) that warrant combined cosmetic and functional septorhinoplasty. The patient's desire for a more attractive or "fashionable" nose is also an important factor. This standard is constantly evolving and is largely dictated by changes in media and fashion.

SURGICAL ACCESS FOR PRIMARY COSMETIC RHINOPLASTY

Common incisions for surgical access in closed and open rhinoplasty are illustrated in **Fig. 2**. The details of the nasal structures are discussed elsewhere in this article. Careful subperichondrial elevation of the soft tissue will provide visualization of the upper and lower lateral cartilages in their passive and unaltered form, and will also minimize postoperative nasal tip hypoesthesia.

Closed Rhinoplasty

Rhinoplasty was traditionally developed as a cosmetic procedure to alter the shape of the nose via a closed (endonasal) surgical access. This technique has survived the test of time and continues to be a principal approach for many surgeons. In the past 3 decades many surgeons have embraced the open rhinoplasty approach via a transcolumellar incision. Both techniques can provide excellent results. However, major differences in surgical technique, training, and visibility are observed between the two approaches. Many surgeons strictly adhere to the open or closed surgical access for all structural deformities. It is the authors' opinion that combination

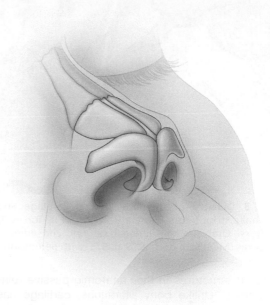

Fig. 2. Common sites of incisions for rhinoplasty. (*From* Bagheri SC, Jo C. Clinical review of oral and maxillofacial surgery. Mosby/Elsevier; 2008. p. 309; with permission.)

of open and closed techniques should dominate the current dictum for modern rhinoplasty surgery Although successful outcomes are achieved via both techniques, when possible students of rhinoplasty should acquire the skills to treat and modify the nose using both methods.

In closed rhinoplasty, the access to the nasal structures is usually via a combination of partial or complete transfixion incisions along with an intercartilagenous (between the lower and upper lateral cartilages) or intracartilagenous (cartilage splitting) incisions. Simultaneous septoplasty or turbinate reduction can be done via separate incisions. The Killian incision can be used for access to the nasal septum when simultaneously using a hemitransfixion incision. The incision is placed at least 5 to 8 mm posterior to the caudal edge of the septal cartilage to avoid compromising the hemitransfixion access. This placement allows surgical access to the cartilaginous and bony nasal dorsum for both reductive and augmentation techniques without direct visualization. The nasal tip and columellar structures can also be modified. The cartilage delivery technique is used to directly visualize and alter the lower lateral cartilage and tip **(Fig. 3)**. The most difficult challenge of the closed rhinoplasty approach is to achieve a predictable and desired alteration of both bony and cartilage structures via minimal direct visualization of

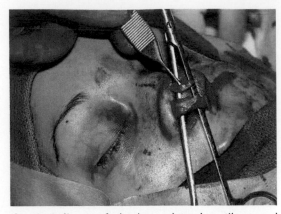

Fig. 3. Delivery of the lower lateral cartilage and cephalic strip. (*From* Fonseca R, Marciani R, Turvey T, editors. Oral and maxillofacial surgery. 2nd edition. St Louis (MO): Saunders; 2009. p. 573; with permission.)

altered structures in their anatomic passive relationships. Unlike bony alterations, cartilage has memory, and maintaining the cartilage in the desired position is difficult, but can be achieved using a variety of cartilage modifications (scoring, transection, repositioning, trimming, sutures, and grafting). Originally the closed technique was predominantly a reductive technique involving dorsal reduction and nasal osteotomies. Nasal tip modification was considered difficult and only amenable to minor changes. Although this remains true, equally complex tip modifications can be done via the closed technique; however, this requires greater training to achieve the surgical comfort and desired final esthetic outcomes. Grafting of the nasal tip structures can be challenging via the closed approach and requires complex understanding of the tip. Graft movement and stability are among the few problems that the surgeon may encounter.

An advantage of the closed rhinoplasty technique is the speed, lesser dissection, and absence of a skin incision. It has been suggested that when compared with closed approach, the open technique (especially without strut grafting) will result in some degree of long-term nasal tip collapse, due to the soft-tissue retraction, scarring, and weakening of the foot plates of the lower lateral cartilages. However, as in many areas of cosmetic surgery, this concept has not been validated by long-term prospective cohort or randomized studies.

An important addition to rhinoplasty surgery was the placement of spreader grafts (see the article by James Koehler elsewhere in this issue for further exploration of this topic) to preserve or increase the nasal valve angle that directly correlates with the respiratory function of the nose. This action can be particularly important with reduction of

the dorsum width. The graft is usually obtained from the nasal septum (or from the ear cartilage), and is positioned between the nasal septum and the upper lateral cartilages on both sides as needed. Spreader grafts can be placed under direct vision and sutured into place using the open technique. However, placement of grafts using the closed approach is more difficult and potentially less stable. A pocket is created by gentle dissection through the intercartilagenous incision between the nasal septum and the upper lateral cartilages bilaterally. The spreader grafts are positioned into the pocket to achieve the desired effect.

In summary, the endonasal or closed rhinoplasty technique is an effective but highly specialized method, especially with respect to complex nasal tip plasty and augmentation. Mastery of this approach is more difficult. The relative difficulty of the closed technique and the more recent emphasis on the open approach in the literature has made this traditional and important method more difficult to master for rising rhinoplasty surgeons. It can be safely hypothesized that closed rhinoplasty surgeons can more easily master the open approach than vice versa.

Open Rhinoplasty

The transcolumellar incision with bilateral marginal extensions, also described as the open rhinoplasty technique, has become progressively popular since the 1980s. This access dramatically facilitates the teaching of rhinoplasty, and significantly contributes to predictable nasal structural modifications (**Fig. 4**). The realization of the flap viability and ability to modify and graft cartilage that has been stripped from its supporting perichondrium has contributed to the success of this approach. Prior to its inception, students of rhinoplasty would have had to learn the complex anatomy and surgical modifications of the closed rhinoplasty

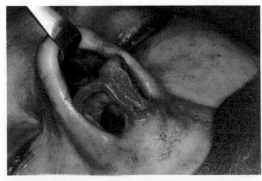

Fig. 4. Exposure of nasal tip using the open rhinoplasty incision.

without visualization of the modified structures, which makes mastery of the technique extremely challenging. The open approach has allowed more rapid understanding of the anatomy by observing students, translating into a greater number of surgeons who acquire the skills and interest for this surgery. This flap allows the placement of complex grafts (shield, columella, tip, supra tip, ala, spreader, and so forth) under direct vision. Although many experienced surgeons may be able to achieve exceptional results and grafting via the closed approach, characteristically this requires a prolonged and sustained learning curve, years of trial and error that may only be achieved later in one's surgical career. The accelerated learning of nasal modifications via the open approach is a great advantage to learning surgeons and their patients.

The greater visibility of the open rhinoplasty also facilitates soft-tissue modification of the nasal tip. In patients with a bulbous nasal tip secondary to an excessively fibrofatty subcutaneous plane, the flap allows direct access to the underlying tissue for careful removal. In these patients the modifications of the cartilagenous structures can be significantly masked by an excessively thick S-STE. Although uncommon, care should be taken not to thin this tissue in excess, which can result in tip dehiscence. Placement of spreader grafts is also greatly facilitated and more accurately performed using the open approach.

Concomitant septoplasty is frequently performed in the patient undergoing primary open rhinoplasty. The septal cartilage is approached for function (deviated septum) or used as a donor site for cartilage reconstruction for the tip, ala, columellar strut, or spreader grafts. Traditionally the septal cartilage is accessed using an endonasal incision (eg, Killian, transfixion). The septal cartilage can also be approached via the open technique for septoplasty or cartilage harvest. As with the endonasal approach, care must be taken to maintain a minimum of 1 cm dorsal and caudal cartilage for preservation of dorsal support. Collapse of this cartilage can result in the saddle-nose deformity. The open approach provides excellent access to the cartilage using a subperichondrial dissection of the septal cartilage from above down to the nasal crest of the maxilla. The cartilage can be easily harvested, modified, and repositioned back to its original location.

The open access also allows direct visualization of the nasal bones. While most reductive nasal modifications can be done via endonasal access, reconstruction and augmentation of the bony and cartilagenous dorsum using autologous (rib, iliac crest) or alloplastic material is greatly facilitated. In summary, rhinoplasty has traditionally been a reductive procedure. The open approach has both facilitated the learning curve for this procedure and enhanced surgeons' ability for addition, reduction, and complex reconstruction of the S-STE as well as bony and cartilagenous structures under direct vision.

Dias advantages of the open rhinoplasty technique include the slight increased operative time for flap elevation, the presence of the transcolumellar scar, and paresthesia of the nasal tip. The scar is usually well concealed under the nasal tip and is not visible on frontal view. The inverted-V transcolumellar incision allows proper alignment of the flap at closure, and also helps camouflage the scar. Surgeons should consider the possibility of keloid formation, especially in African American patients with a prior history. Paresthesia (hypoesthesia or anesthesia) of the nasal tip is common, especially after debulking of the underlying S-STE, and can persist for more than 1 year postoperatively. Strict adherence to the subperichondrial plane and, when possible, decreasing the disruption of the flap, can minimize this postoperative sequela. However, all patients should be informed about the possibility of prolonged nasal tip paresthesia.

TREATMENT PLAN
Specific Surgical Techniques

Although further detailed description of surgical maneuvers for rhinoplasty are discussed elsewhere in this issue, here the authors briefly describe some of the basic strategies for modification of the 4 anatomic regions of the nose (radix, dorsum, tip, nasal base) as related to primary rhinoplasty. These regions are also summarized in **Table 2**.

Radix Modification

The majority of radix modifications involve reduction or augmentation. Reduction has to be done in harmony with dorsal and tip modifications, and this is generally achieved using a rasp or osteotomes via a closed or open access. The radix has to be balanced to match the dorsum. Reduction of the radix alone will further enhance the projection of the nasal dorsum. Augmentation procedures have been done on this area since the 1930s. Many materials have been used for this purpose, including septal or conchal cartilage, dermis, fascia, and bone. The authors prefer the use of either temporalis fascia or acellular donated human dermis (alloderm). The temporalis fascia can be easily harvested via a temporal incision within the hairline. The graft is subsequently

Table 2
Basic strategies for modification of the 4 anatomic regions of the nose (radix, dorsum, tip, nasal base) as related to primary rhinoplasty

RADIX	
Reduction	Rasp or osteotomy via open or closed techniques
Augmentation	Can be done with alloplastic (eg, alloderm) or autologous material (bone, cartilage, fascia)
DORSUM	
Reduction	Width reduction with combination of lateral and medial osteotomies. Profile reduction with rasp or osteotome
	Excessive dorsal reduction will likely require bilateral nasal osteotomies for closure of open book deformities
	Spreader grafts should be considered to maintain the nasal valve angle for preservation of airflow
Augmentation	Can be done with alloplastic (eg, alloderm) or autologous material (bone, cartilage, fascia)
	Bony and cartilagenous augmentation can be done simultaneously
TIP	
Elevation	Columellar strut, shield, and/or tip graft, suturing to nasal septum
Volume reduction	Cartilage excision or trim. Dome and tip defining sutures
Definition	Combination of sutures, grafts, and cartilage excision or trim
Projection	Graft, suture (dorsal reduction will also affect projection)
BASE	
Nostril	Reduction in size is done using nostril sill excision, and nasal flare and alar base is reduced with alar wedge excision
Ala	Graft to alter alar shape and contour
Columella	Excision or graft

inserted at the radix on completion of the rhinoplasty, using an attached needle that is pulled through at the nasion point (**Fig. 5**). Overgrafting by 25% to 30% is recommended to account for subsequent graft resorption and atrophy.

Dorsum Modification

Traditional rhinoplasty surgeons alter the dorsum to match the esthetics of the nasal tip. Modern rhinoplasty techniques emphasize the concept of a balanced nose, whereby reduction and augmentation strategies are used to achieve harmony between all components, thus achieving the ideal height of the dorsum. Alterations of the nasal dorsum or the osseocartilagenous vault are complex, and involve both cosmetic and functional factors. Reduction of the dorsum is usually done by rasp or osteotomes (**Fig. 6**). The cartilagenous (upper lateral and septal cartilages) can be excised with a scalpel or scissors. Depending on the extent

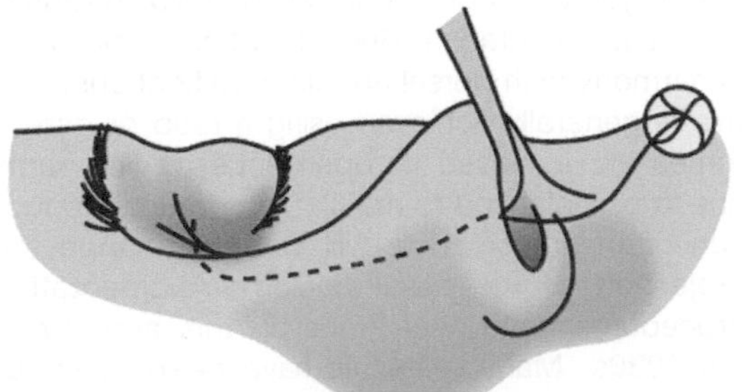

Fig. 5. Diagram of radix augmentation using alloderm or temporalis fascia. (*From* Bagheri SC, Bell RB, Khan HA, editors. Current therapy in oral and maxillofacial surgery. St Louis (MO): Mosby/Elsevier; 2012. p. 897; with permission.)

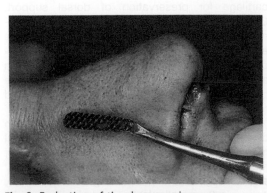

Fig. 6. Reduction of the dorsum using a rasp.

of reduction, an open-book deformity may result that can be addressed using lateral nasal osteotomies. Narrowing of the nasal vault will affect the internal nasal valve angle. Spreader grafts can be used to prevent this complication. The combination of simultaneous medial and lateral osteotomies are less frequently used because of the difficulty in controlling the mediolateral position of the nasal bone. Lateral nasal osteotomies are also used to decrease the width of the dorsum. These osteotomies are best conducted through a small endonasal incision at the inferior and lateral aspect of the piriform rim. However, some surgeons prefer to do this via a small transcutaneous stab incision. A thermoplastic nasal splint is used after nasal osteotomies to stabilize the segments, and is kept in place for 1 to 2 weeks (**Fig. 7**).

Dorsal augmentation can be achieved using allogenic or alloplastic material. Septal and ear cartilage can be used for minor augmentation in conjunction with fascia or acellular dermal grafts. Major dorsal reconstruction is best achieved with rib (cartilage and bone) or iliac crest. Alloplastic material such as silicone or porous polyethylene (Medpore) is less frequently used because of frequent postoperative complications (graft movement, infection, dehiscence).

Tip Modification

Nasal tip surgery is the most difficult and challenging part of cosmetic rhinoplasty. Adherence to sound surgical techniques and emphasis on minor tip changes allows for a more controlled outcome. The nasal tip can be analyzed by 6 characteristics: volume (based on size of lateral crura), width (interdomal distance), shape (broad, bulbous, boxy), projection, rotation, and definition. These characteristics are interrelated and are not strictly independently modified (eg, cephalic lateral crura resection is primarily done to reduce the tip volume, but it also increases projection

and alters the definition). Understanding of this allows the surgeon to better visualize the final outcome. Surgical treatment plans that alter the tip are designed to modify these characteristics. A complete discussion of these techniques is beyond the scope of this article, and the reader should refer to the suggested readings for further study. However, basic modifications for each characteristic are summarized in **Table 3**.

Nasal Base Modification

When indicated, nasal base modifications should be an integral part of primary cosmetic rhinoplasty. This area is complex and integrates anatomically with the alar base, nostril openings, external nasal valve, columella, and tip. The vast majority of alar base modifications include an alar base wedge excision, a nostril sill/floor excision, or both (**Fig. 8**). The resulting scar is well concealed and infrequently causes any complications. The nostril sill excision is extended into the floor of the nose, and can be used to reduce the size and visibility of the nostril floor on frontal view. The alar wedge excision is made in a curvilinear fashion just superior to the alar crease. This excision will reduce the alar flare, and is commonly used in African American rhinoplasty. The two incisions can be combined to achieve reduction in alar flare and nostril size. The intraoral alar cinch procedure can also be used to reduce the alar width.

Grafts

Grafting is an important part of modern rhinoplasty. Multiple autogenous donor sites and

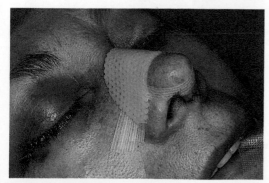
Fig. 7. Thermoplastic nasal splint is used after nasal osteotomies to stabilize the segments.

Table 3
Nasal tip characteristics and basic surgical modifications

Characteristic	Primary Modification Technique
Volume	Reduction: cephalic lateral crura resection Augmentation: shield graft
Width	Reduction: interdomal sutures
Definition	Domal equalization sutures, domal definition sutures, domal creation sutures
Projection	Tip graft, projection suture, columellar strut
Rotation	Rotation suture (to nasal septum), columellar strut, tip graft
Shape	Graft (tip, ala), cartilage excision/trim, sutures

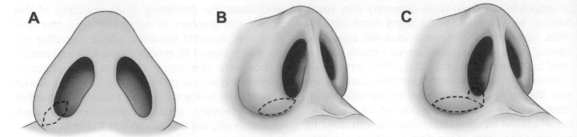

Fig. 8. (*A*) Excision of the nostril sill. (*B*) Alar wedge excision. (*C*) Combined sill/alar excision. (*From* Daniel RK. Rhinoplasty: an atlas of surgical techniques. New York: Springer; 2002; with permission.)

several alloplastic grafting materials are available. Most current rhinoplasty surgeons use autogenous cartilage grafts for the majority of primary cosmetic rhinoplasties.

Septal cartilage is the primary choice for most tip, columella, alar, and dorsal cartilage grafting. In cases where the septal cartilage is not available (previous septoplasty or secondary rhinoplasty), the concha can be easily harvested. Temporalis fascia and decellularized human dermis (Alloderm) are commonly used grafts for radix or other soft-tissue grafting.

Fig. 9 shows the preoperative and postoperative appearance of patient who underwent cosmetic rhinoplasty and caudal septoplasty. The surgical procedure included dorsal reduction and tip plasty (cephalic lateral crural resection, interdomal and tip-defining sutures). Lateral osteotomies were not conducted on this patient to maintain the balance between the tip and dorsal width. **Fig. 10** shows preoperative and

postoperative views of a younger patient who underwent a similar procedure that also included tip grafting.

POSTOPERATIVE CARE

Routine postoperative care of the rhinoplasty patient should address analgesia, nausea, nutrition, antimicrobials, nasal hygiene, swelling, possible epistaxis and, most importantly, postoperative visits and support of the patient during the healing process. The authors advocate frequent postoperative visits not only to re-enforce wound healing but also for emotional support, especially with respect to the facial edema seen during the immediate postoperative period.

The patient should be instructed to rest in bed with the head elevated, with frequent application of gentle cold compress for the first 24 hours when possible to reduce edema. White gauze is taped or suspended at the nostrils to minimize

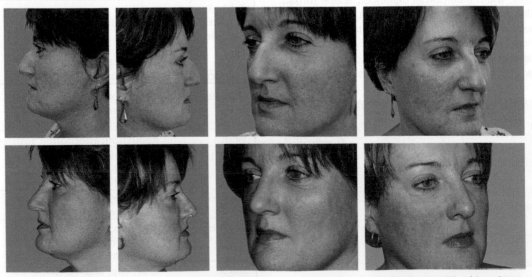

Fig. 9. Preoperative and postoperative photographs of a patients who underwent cosmetic rhinoplasty and caudal septoplasty.

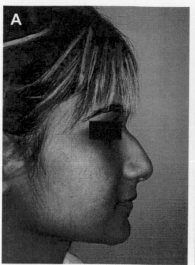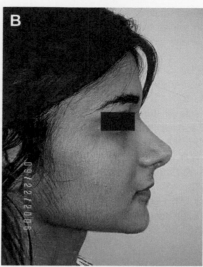

Fig. 10. (*A*) Preoperative and (*B*) postoperative views of a younger patient who underwent a similar procedure to the patient in **Fig. 9**, but which also included tip grafting.

dripping of blood. Although significant postoperative hemorrhage is uncommon, most patients will have minor epistaxis (especially with nasal osteotomies). Intranasal packings can accumulate blood clots and mucous secretions, and can significantly contribute to postoperative discomfort and pain. The intranasal septal packings/splints are sutured to the membranous septum to avoid displacement deeper into the nostril. The authors recommend placing the suture tie at an anterior and visible location for ease of removal.

Patients are encouraged to ambulate early and not to remain in bed. This action will help minimize edema, and reduce postoperative pulmonary complications and deep venous thrombosis. The nostrils can be gently cleansed with normal saline and coated with petroleum jelly. The sutures are removed at 7 to 9 days postoperatively. Many patients present with significant anxiety related to the postoperative visit (removal of sutures or intranasal splints), and may require encouragement and support. Intravenous sedation can be used in select patients for reduction of anxiety, complete suctioning of the nasal cavity, and removal of old blood clots and sutures. In cases of nasal osteotomies, the nasal cast is removed at 7 to 14 days. The patient is advised to avoid contact with the nasal structures. Postoperative systemic steroids can be used to reduce edema, although this may not be indicated in all patients. Steroids (triamcinolone) can be injected into the nasal tip in cases of prolonged nasal tip edema. The authors recommend at least 3 injections at 1-week intervals. Similarly, irregularities and depressions can be addressed with injectable fillers after several months have passed. Unfavorable results should be immediately addressed and acknowledged. Unless there are grossly abnormal findings, enough time should elapse before any revision rhinoplasty is considered (discussed elsewhere in this article).

SUGGESTED READINGS

Adamson P, Smith O, Cole P. The effect of cosmetic rhinoplasty on nasal patency. Laryngoscope 1990; 100:357.

Anderson JR, Ries WR. Rhinoplasty: emphasizing the external approach. New York: Thieme Inc; 1986.

Bagheri SC, Khan HA. Current trends in rhinoplasty. In: Bagheri SC, Bell RB, Khan HA, editors. Current therapy in oral and maxillofacial surgery. St Louis (MO): Mosby/Elsevier; 2012.

Bagheri SC, Khan HA, Jahangirian A, Rad S, Mortazavi H. An analysis of 101 primary cosmetic Rhinoplasty. J Oral Maxillofac Surg June 2011. [Epub ahead of print].

Constantian M. Four common anatomic variants that predispose to unfavorable rhinoplasty results. Plast Reconstr Surg 2000;105:316.

Constantinides M, Adamson PA, Cole P. The long term effects of open cosmetic septorhinoplasty on nasal air flow. Arch Otolaryngol Head Neck Surg 1996; 122:44.

Daniel RK. Rhinoplasty: an atlas of surgical techniques. New York: Springer; 2002.

Galdino GM, DaSilva And D, Gunter JP. Digital photography for rhinoplasty. Plast Reconstr Surg 2002; 109(4):1421–34.

Gandomi B, Bayat A, Kazemei T. Outcomes of septo-plasty in young adults: the nasal obstruction septo-plasty effectiveness study. Am J Otolaryngol 2010; 31(3):189–92.

Gunter JP, Rohrich RJ. Correction of the pinched nasal tip with alar spreader grafts. Plast Reconstr Surg 2003;112:1533–9.

Gunter JP. The merits of the open approach in rhino-plasty. Plast Reconstr Surg 1997;99(3):863–7.

Johnson CM, Toriumi DM. Open structure rhinoplasty. Philadelphia: W.B. Sauders; 1990.

Rohrich RJ, Bolden K. Ethnic rhinoplasty. Clin Plast Surg 2010;37:353–70.

Rohrich RJ, Hollier LH. Use of spreader grafts in the external approach to rhinoplasty. Clin Plast Surg 1996;23:255–62.

Sheen JH. Spreader graft: a method of reconstructing the roof of the middle nasal vault following rhino-plasty. Plast Reconstr Surg 1984;73:230–9.

Simons RL. A personal report: emphasizing the endo-nasal approach. Facial Plast Surg Clin North Am 2004;12(1):15–34.

Tardy ME Jr, Dayan S, Hecht D. Preoperative rhinoplasty: evaluation and analysis. Otolaryngol Clin North Am 2002;35:1.

Tebbetts JB. Rethinking the logic and techniques of primary tip rhinoplasty. Clin Plast Surg 1996;23:245.

Toriumi DM, Pero CD. Asian rhinoplasty. Clin Plast Surg 2010;37:335–52.

Toriumi D, Mueller R, Grosch T. Vascular anatomy of the nose and the external rhinoplasty approach. Arch Otolaryngol Head Neck Surg 1996;122:24.

Septoplasty in Conjunction with Cosmetic Rhinoplasty

Carey J. Nease, MD*, R. Chad Deal, MD

KEYWORDS

- Septoplasty • Rhinoplasty • Cosmetic rhinoplasty
- Nasal septum

In 1908, Frank Lloyd Wright said, "Form follows function—that has been misunderstood. Form and function should be one, joined in a spiritual union." It is the purpose of this article to discuss the intimate relationship that the form of the nasal septum and the esthetics of the nose have with one another and that alterations of either can significantly affect the other. Surgeons from several specialties perform surgical alterations of the external and internal nose, including head and neck surgeons, oral and maxillofacial surgeons, cosmetic surgeons, and plastic and reconstructive surgeons; however, many of the advancements in nasal reconstruction, functional improvement, and cosmetic improvement have been kept within the literature of their respective fields. For obvious reasons it would be wise for rhinoplasty surgeons, regardless of their background and training, to have a solid understanding of the form and function of the nose so that they may bridge the gaps of their specialty and provide the best possible outcome for their patients.

HISTORICAL SUMMARY OF SEPTOPLASTY

Likely, an Egyptian physician named Ni-Ankh Sekhmet, who removed a nasal polyp for King Sahura, performed the first known surgery on the inside of the nose.[1] Unfortunately, most intranasal procedures were slow to progress because of the substantial bleeding associated with the highly vascular anatomy and poor visualization of the structures of interest. It took much advancement in knowledge of nasal anatomy and physiology,

as well as discovery of the use of vasoconstrictors in this area, as described by Rethi, before endonasal surgery became both safe and effective.[2] The first described submucosal approach to the septum was described by Leinhardt, and this concept was advanced by others to describe access to the entire septum to correct deviations.[3]

Most well known for septal surgery was Killian, who put most of this knowledge together and specifically detailed lifting bilateral submucosal windows after using a cocaine-epinephrine solution. He described following this with a fairly aggressive resection of both septal cartilage and bone. Killian was very precise in his recommendations for the location of the incision to leave support to the nasal dorsum and tip and described preserving both dorsal and caudal support to prevent collapse.[3]

After Killian, the most notable advancements came from Cottle, who described elevation of the mucoperichondrium on only one side. This was a major advancement because up to this point septal surgery was plagued with complications associated with the damage of the nasal mucosa and loss of support from overresection.[3] Meanwhile, advancements in the reconstructive and esthetic aspects of nasal surgery have taken place on their own timeline, which is discussed elsewhere. As further knowledge has been gained in the anatomy, physiology, and surgical techniques of all aspects related to internal and external nasal surgery, most have come to the conclusion that they are indeed inseparable. A good rhinoplasty surgeon should also be a competent septoplasty

Southern Surgical Arts, 200 Manufacturer's Road, Chattanooga, TN 37405, USA
* Corresponding author.
E-mail address: drnease@southernsurgicalarts.com

Oral Maxillofacial Surg Clin N Am 24 (2012) 49–58
doi:10.1016/j.coms.2011.10.006

surgeon. We discuss relevant anatomy, surgical techniques, and possible complications of septoplasty surgery and how it relates to cosmetic rhinoplasty.

RELEVANT NASAL SEPTAL ANATOMY

For the purposes of this article, it is important to understand a brief overview of the external nasal anatomy, related axial directions, and their corresponding nomenclature (**Fig. 1**). The nasal septum is composed of both bony and cartilaginous portions that each deserve specific consideration and have unique importance (**Fig. 2**). The anatomic relationships of the cartilage and bony segments of the septum become critical both in incision selection and approach to the septum. When performing a septoplasty for the removal of cartilage or bone for correction of deviations or for the harvest of grafting material, several techniques have been used over the years.

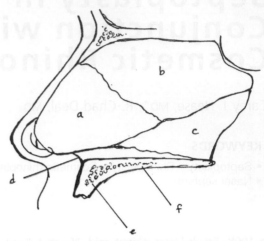

Fig. 2. Nasal septum, sagittal view. (a) Quadrangular cartilage. (b) Perpendicular plate of the ethmoid bone. (c) Vomer (bone). (d) Anterior nasal spine. (e) Pre-maxilla. (f) Palatine bone. (*Courtesy of* Carey Nease, MD, Lookout Mountain, Georgia.)

Generally speaking, most nasal surgeons would now say that what you take out is not as important as what you leave behind. Specifically when it comes to support of the nasal dorsum, common thought is that preserving an "L" strut of at least 1.5 cm in the dorsal and caudal areas of the quadrangular cartilaginous septum is adequate.[4] If overresection has occurred, a "saddle nose" deformity can result (**Fig. 3**). Another possibility is collapse of the nasal tip with resultant ptosis, which can lead to a poor esthetic result and also airway obstruction (**Fig. 4**). Preservation of support can be particularly difficult when dealing with the previously operated septum, which is discussed later in this article.

Basic understanding of the anatomic relationship of the dorsal septum and the upper lateral cartilages is critical for preserving the patency of the internal nasal valve and thus the anterior aspect of the nasal airway. This particular region of the nasal airway has a significant impact on the airflow through the nasal passages, which reinforces the point that septoplasty and rhinoplasty surgery do significantly affect one another. Maintenance of adequate nasal airflow should never be compromised and thus should be a consideration when performing any nasal surgery (**Fig. 5**). It is also important to recognize that other internal nasal structures, such as the inferior turbinate, can also affect nasal airflow. The septo/rhinoplasty surgeon should be able to diagnose a hypertrophied inferior turbinate and should also be comfortable addressing the pathology at the time of a septo/rhinoplasty procedure (**Fig. 6**).

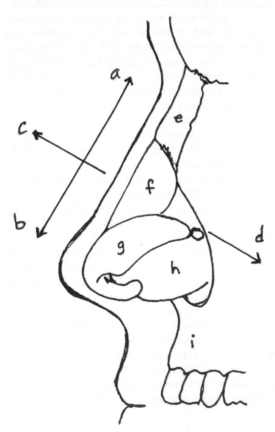

Fig. 1. External nasal anatomy and axial nomenclature. (a) Cephalic (cranial). (b) Caudal. (c) Anterior (dorsal). (d) Posterior. (e) Nasal bones. (f) Upper lateral cartilage. (g) Lower lateral cartilage. (h) Cartilaginous septum. (i) Pre-maxilla. (*Courtesy of* Carey Nease, MD, Lookout Mountain, Georgia.)

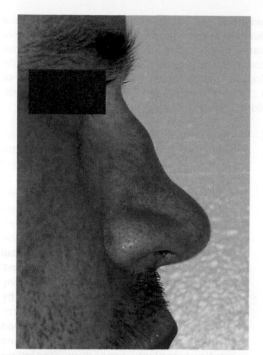

Fig. 3. Saddle nose deformity. Common result from lack of septal support or surgical overresection of septal cartilage.

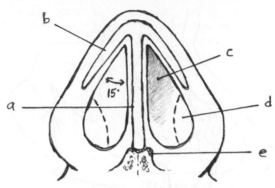

Fig. 5. Basal view of the internal nasal valve with cross-sectional anatomy. (a) Cartilaginous septum. (b) Upper lateral cartilage. (c) Airway at the internal nasal valve. (d) Inferior turbinate. (e) Maxillary crest (bone). (*Courtesy of* Carey Nease, MD, Lookout Mountain, Georgia.)

It is also important for the rhinoplasty surgeon to understand the concentration of arterial blood supply that exists in the anterior septal region, for both hemostasis considerations and flap survival after septoplasty (**Fig. 7**). Most of the blood supply to the anterior septum comes from 3 distinct arteries: the superior labial, greater palatine, and anterior ethmoidal vessels. These 3 arteries come together in the anterior septum to form a region known as Kiesselbach plexus. This anatomy is important to the septo/rhinoplasty surgeon because it is the area in which most of the operation will take place. Regarding the posterior septum, the sphenopalatine and posterior ethmoidal arteries are responsible for most of the blood supply (See **Fig. 7**). Only in certain situations, such as a high posterior bony deflection, should this anatomy be encountered. Inadvertent damage to the sphenopalatine vessels in particular can cause brisk arterial bleeding that is difficult to control and may require more expertise,

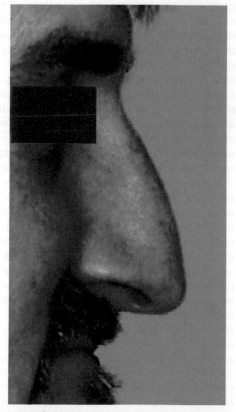

Fig. 4. Nasal tip ptosis.

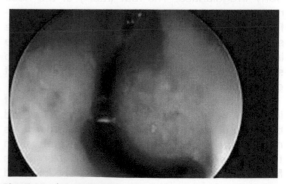

Fig. 6. Endoscopic view of left nasal passage showing nasal septum and enlarged inferior turbinate.

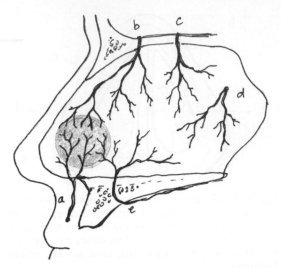

Fig. 7. Blood supply of the nasal septum. (a) Superior labial artery. (b) Anterior ethmoidal artery. (c) Posterior ethmoidal artery. (d) Sphenopalatine artery. (e) Greater palatine artery. Shaded area represents Kiesselbach plexus of the anterior septum. (*Courtesy of Carey Nease, MD, Lookout Mountain, Georgia.*)

such as posterior nasal packing or even interventional radiology consultation for embolization.

INDICATIONS FOR SEPTOPLASTY WITH COSMETIC RHINOPLASTY

There are several indications for combining a septoplasty with a cosmetic rhinoplasty that can be both functional and esthetic in nature. Commonly, the techniques for tip support preservation after either an open or endonasal rhinoplasty require having a cartilage strut graft available for placement between the medial crura. Further, if tip definition is needed, a shield graft may be warranted. Less often, the dorsum of the nose may need grafting for augmentation or camouflage of bony irregularities. The root (radix) of the nose may also need to be addressed to fill a deep nasofrontal angle. Finally, other useful grafts include spreader grafts to assist in widening an acute internal nasal valve and batten onlay grafts to support the nasal ala sidewalls and prevent collapse of the external nasal valve.

All of these needs can be supplied fully, or at least primarily, from the harvest of cartilage and bone from the nasal septum. If the septum does not provide enough material, cartilage grafts from the ears or ribs may also be harvested. Temporalis fascia is also easily accessible and provides good soft tissue for dorsal coverage and augmentation. The list of reasons to perform septoplasty is

extensive but most commonly includes septal deviation with obstruction, bone spurs, nasal valve pathology, or the "crooked nose" from either congenital or traumatic causes. All of these conditions can and should be treated at the time of a cosmetic rhinoplasty. These are discussed individually in the following paragraphs.

1. Nasal obstruction: most commonly caused by deflection of the cartilaginous portion of the nasal septum, which will lead to a unilateral narrowing of the internal nasal valve region in the anterior nasal airway. Even what seems a very trivial deflection of the cartilaginous septum in this region can cause significant symptoms of obstruction. Other less common causes of obstruction would include nasal polyps, inferior turbinate hypertrophy, external valve collapse, and other nasal masses. Any polyp or mass should have its own workup by a specialist and should be addressed according its characteristics. These problems, when present, should be addressed before any cosmetic rhinoplasty procedure. Regarding inferior turbinate hypertrophy, it is in the authors' opinion that the most effective treatment is submucosal resection of the excess bone and soft tissue in the anterior one-third of the turbinate with preservation of the mucosa. Again, unless the rhinoplasty surgeon is comfortable with treatment of these issues, the patient should be referred to a specialist and treated accordingly.

2. Internal nasal valve pathology: this can be caused by both congenital pathology and traumatic/surgical deformities. Congenitally, a weak upper lateral cartilage and/or weakness of the ala of the lower lateral cartilages can cause collapse on inspiration. The internal valve region can also be compromised by septal deviation or a congenitally narrow nasal valve from an overprojected and narrow dorsum. Internal nasal valve pathology can also be iatrogenic from overresection of the lower lateral cartilages or separation of the upper lateral cartilage from the dorsal septum, with resultant scarring and narrowing of the angle itself. Most problems in this area can be avoided with preservation of cartilage support and with minimal disturbance of the native anatomy.

3. Bone spurs: these deformities of the bony septum are commonly located inferiorly as a lateral extension of the vomer into the inferior aspect of the nasal airway. This is less commonly a cause of an obstruction and may be asymptomatic. A common symptom of a bony nasal spur is a headache that derives

from the spur making contact with the inferior turbinate or lateral nasal sidewall. When a bony spur is observed at the time of septoplasty, it should be removed. Removal can be down through any of the described approaches to the septum and should be done with a through-cutting forceps to prevent inadvertent fracture of the cribriform plate superiorly, leading to leakage of cerebrospinal fluid (CSF). Bone spurs can also come directly off of the maxillary crest and obstruct the airway along the nasal floor (**Fig. 8**).

4. Harvest of cartilage and/or bone: as noted previously, there are several reasons, both functional and esthetic, that may require harvesting of septal cartilage. Strut and shield grafts, spreader grafts, batten grafts, dorsal onlay grafts, and radix grafts are those most commonly used. "Crushed" cartilage has several uses, including camouflaging irregularities throughout the nose or as a plumping graft on the anterior nasal spine to increase the nasolabial angle. The standard harvest of septal cartilage, when no pathology exists, is best approached through a Killian incision in the authors' opinion (**Fig. 9**). This approach is recommended to avoid loss of any tip support and can be combined with an external or endonasal rhinoplasty for minimal risk of complications. Steps in approach and harvest are listed later in this article. If the septal cartilage has been previously harvested and more cartilage is needed, the next best source is the conchal cartilage of the external ear. Preoperatively, if there is reasonable suspicion that this

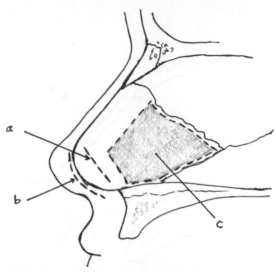

Fig. 9. Sagittal view showing endonasal surgical approaches for septoplasty. (a) Killian incision. (b) Hemitransfixion incision (along caudal border of cartilaginous septum). (c) Shaded area represents typical harvested section for grafting. Note: When a full transfixion incision is desired to de-project the tip, the dissection of the septum can be performed through an incision in the same location in the membranous septum as that of the hemitransfixion type. (*Courtesy of* Carey Nease, MD, Lookout Mountain, Georgia.)

will be required, the ear should be prepped and draped. Other sources of cartilage or bone are the anterior sixth to seventh rib, and, if available, cadaveric sources. Calvarial bone from the outer cortex is also rarely used but may be required when there is near total collapse of the nose and rib cartilage is unavailable. If soft tissue is needed for a dorsal graft, the temporalis fascia remains the preferred source and is easily accessible through a postauricular incision.

5. Crooked nose: as mentioned previously, the crooked nose can be the result of either a congenital anomaly or traumatic deformity. In these cases, there will almost always be a septal deformity as well. The approach to correction of the crooked nose should therefore always address the septum. Whether a crooked nose is congenital or traumatic, the septum can be deformed in several ways[3] (**Fig. 10**). A significantly deviated dorsal septum is best approached and corrected through an external approach. Separation of the external upper and lateral cartilages from the dorsal septum and elevation of bilateral mucoperichondrial flaps is the first step in the procedure. This

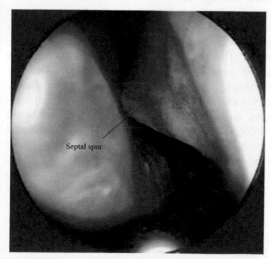

Fig. 8. Endoscopic view of the right nasal passage near the floor of the nose showing bony septal spur touching the inferior turbinate.

Septal spur

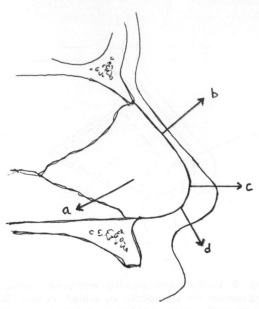

Fig. 10. Common septal cartilage deformities affecting the shape of the external nose. (a) Cartilaginous septal deflection. (b) Dorsal hump, tension nose, or saddle nose. (c) Tip characteristics: Underrotated or overrotated, underprojected or overprojected, tip ptosis. (d) Elongated caudal septum causing hanging columella and vestibular show; subluxation of caudal septum causing nostril asymmetry. (*Courtesy of* Carey Nease, MD, Lookout Mountain, Georgia.)

then allows excellent access and visualization of the deflected cartilage. Repair of the deformity can be accomplished through cartilage removal, scoring, and/or cartilage onlay grafts. When the septal deflection is difficult to straighten, an oppositely deflected piece of harvested cartilage can be sewn onto the native dorsal septum with mattress sutures to balance the bend. A combination of techniques may be warranted, and investigators differ on preferred techniques. Once the septum has been addressed, other steps may be taken to straighten the "crooked" nose, including, but not limited to, medial and lateral osteotomies and internally and externally placed splints.

OPERATIVE APPROACH TO THE NASAL SEPTUM

The approach to septoplasty is variable based on goals, severity of deformity, and the surgeon's preference and experience. Options include a Killian incision, hemitransfixion, full transfixion, and an external approach. An endoscopic approach is also an option but is beyond the scope of this article.

The Killian incision is particularly beneficial because it preserves the tip support mechanisms of the caudal septum, and specifically the medial crural footplate attachment to the caudal septum. With this approach, harvesting of cartilage and bone for grafting or removing bone spurs or correcting a mild septal deviation is easily accomplished while preserving nasal support. The concept of support preservation was described first by Cottle in 1948 as an alternative to Killian's more aggressive resection techniques. His teachings are widely accepted by nasal surgeons today. The mucoperichondrial flap is often elevated on only one side when performing the Killian incision. This is different from the original "Killian septoplasty," which described bilateral flap elevation and significant cartilage and bony removal.[3] A hemitransfixion incision is located at the caudal end of the septum, which provides access to the caudal cartilage to allow correction of deflections at this point and also access to anterior nasal spine if necessary. This is commonly accomplished with bilateral flap elevation for wide access to the cartilaginous and bony septum. For this reason, it is very suitable for harvest of cartilage and bone, removal of bony spurs, and repair of a dorsal or caudal cartilaginous deflection from an endonasal approach. Methods of repair include cartilage scoring, suturing techniques, and cartilage onlay grafts to straighten the septum. All of these techniques are possible with the hemitransfixion incision. A full transfixion incision is an extension of the hemitransfixion incision, with the addition of complete release of the medial crural footplates from the caudal septum. This is desirable when de-projecting the nasal tip is indicated from an esthetic perspective.

All of the aforementioned techniques can be done through an internal (endonasal) approach (see **Fig. 9**). For more direct and extensive access to the dorsal septum, an external approach can be performed at the time of an open rhinoplasty technique. This approach requires separation of the upper lateral cartilages from the dorsal septal cartilage. This provides the most substantial view of the entire septum, and all of the septal pathologies and harvesting needs can be addressed through this approach (**Fig. 11**). The potential downside to this approach is potential scarring of the superior portion of the internal nasal valve that may lead to narrowing the angle and causing nasal obstruction. Corrections of internal nasal valve deformities are discussed later in this article.

DESCRIPTION OF SEPTOPLASTY PROCEDURE STEPS

1. Betadine preparation of nasal vestibules and external nose and cheeks; trim vibrissae.[5]

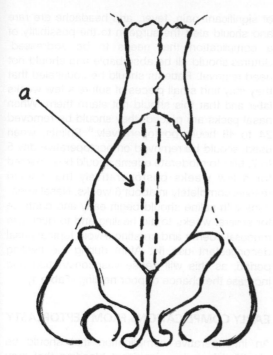

Fig. 11. (Un-roofed) Frontal view of an external approach to septoplasty. (a) Dashed lines represent incision separating the upper lateral cartilage from the cartilaginous septum providing access to the entire septum and thus excellent visualization. (*Courtesy of* Carey Nease, MD, Lookout Mountain, Georgia.)

2. Inject the septum, bilaterally, both anteriorly and posteriorly, with 1% lidocaine with epinephrine 1:100,000 to hydro-dissect the mucoperichondrial flaps and until a blanching of the mucosa is noted. Typically about 15 mL total is needed. Wait 5 to 10 minutes for vasoconstriction. Apply topical oxymetazoline or phenylephrine on cotton pledgets for additional vasoconstriction and inferior turbinate size reduction (will improve visualization).
3. Retract the columella with a small nasal speculum to expose the caudal margin of the septum.
4. Make a Killian or hemitransfixion incision along the caudal border of the cartilaginous septum with a no. 15 blade. A hemitransfixion incision extending from the anterior septal angle to the posterior septal angle is used to gain access to the caudal septum. A Killian incision can be used if access to the caudal septum is not necessary.
5. With a no. 15 blade, incise the perichondrium of the septum adjacent to the caudal septum

on one side. The author (CJN) prefers the left as he is right handed; a left-sided approach was described by Killian as well.[3]

6. Perform a subperichondrial dissection with a Freer or Cottle elevator along the lower half of the anterior septum to allow harvesting of septal cartilage. Do not extend this dissection too high, so that later in the dissection a precise pocket tunnel can be made to place a spreader graft via an endonasal approach, if indicated, and to preserve dorsal support.
7. Repeat maneuver 5 on the opposite side of the septum in the case of a hemitransfixion incision.
8. Remove a window of quadrangular cartilage inferiorly and posteriorly, preserving a dorsal and caudal strut of at least 1.5 cm to provide sufficient support. Place the cartilage in saline on the back table for use later in the case. A segment of the ethmoid bone can be removed at this time as well, and should be done with double-action scissors or through-cutting forceps. Avoid high resection or overmanipulation of the bone, as doing so may lead to fracture of the cribriform plate and a CSF leak.
9. If the caudal septum needs shortening, it may be done at this step in the procedure via direct excision of 1 to 3 mm in a vertical fashion with a no. 15 blade.
10. Irrigate the space between the flaps with saline and ensure hemostasis, then suture the flaps together in a quilting fashion with a 4-0 plain gut suture on a straight (Keith) needle. Close the anterior mucosal incision with either 4-0 chromic or plain gut suture.
11. In some cases, silastic splints may be indicated, especially in instances where large areas of cartilage and bone were removed. The splints should be removed in 5 to 7 days.
12. If packs are desired, they are placed at the completion of the case and removed 24 to 48 hours postoperatively. Some investigators believe that nasal packing use postoperatively can improve subjective breathing long term and also potentially lower the risk for residual deviations of the septum.[6]

COSMETIC INDICATIONS FOR SEPTOPLASTY: THE HANGING COLUMELLA AND TENSION NOSE

A hanging columella, which describes the excess columellar show on profile view, can be addressed through an endonasal incision at the caudal end of the cartilaginous septum. The normal appearance of the alar-columellar relationship should be 2 to 4 mm. Often, the caudal septum will need to be resected by 1 to 3 mm, and a strip of overlying mucosa may need to be removed as well. Closure of this defect, along with suturing of the medial crural footplates to the septum's free edge, will repair the hanging columella by repositioning it posteriorly.[7] A tension nose results from an overly prominent cartilaginous dorsum that creates a tent-pole appearance to the supratip region of the lower dorsum. This is corrected by lowering of the dorsal septal cartilage and can be accomplished easily through either an external or endonasal approach. When more extensive tip surgery is required, however, the external approach is preferred.[8] The amount to be removed depends on the esthetic appearance of the dorsum, and is adequate when a slight supratip break is present. Excess removal can result in loss of tip support, a "scooped" look, and possibly even a saddle nose deformity.

REOPERATIVE CONSIDERATIONS

The previously operated septum presents several potential problems. Most importantly to the cosmetic rhinoplasty surgeon is that the needed cartilage and/or bone for grafting will be limited by what was left behind by the previous surgeon. For this reason, the patient should be aware that a harvest of ear or rib cartilage is a possibility. Besides harvesting concerns, adhesions between the flaps may make elevation of the flaps difficult and increase the likelihood of perforation. Blood supply to the septum in the previously operated areas will also be compromised to some extent, also placing the patient at higher risk for poor healing and late septal perforations. It is in the authors' experience that a previously operated septum is best approached through a transfixion-type incision with elevation of both flaps with slow, careful dissection. If it becomes obvious that either the donor qualities of the septum are poor and/or the scarring is so severe that the mucous membranes are tearing in several places, then one should abort the septoplasty sooner rather than later. External approaches are also appropriate in this circumstance when combined with external rhinoplasty for excellent visualization of the entire septum.

POSTOPERATIVE MANAGEMENT

In addition to the usual concerns that should be in the back of the mind of the rhinoplasty surgeon, when a septoplasty is performed concurrently there are a few unique considerations. At the follow-up visits, the septum should be carefully inspected for normal healing, a midline position, and absence of a hematoma or infection. The presence

of significant pain, fever, and headache are rare and should alert the surgeon to the possibility of a complication that needs to be addressed. Sutures should all be absorbable and should not need removal. Patients should be counseled that they may find small pieces of suture a few weeks later and that this should not alarm them. When nasal packs are placed, they should be removed 24 to 48 hours postoperatively.[6] Splints, when used, should be removed on postoperative day 5 to 7. Mild to moderate edema should be expected for a few weeks postoperatively that should resolve completely in about 6 weeks. Nasal irrigations with saline should begin early and continue for several weeks to aid healing and to decrease mucosal edema and crusting. Avoid topical nasal decongestant use (ie, Afrin) during the healing period, as this will cause vasoconstriction and increase the chance of poor healing (**Table 1**).

EARLY COMPLICATIONS FROM SEPTOPLASTY

An intraoperative complication that should be identified includes significant bleeding that may require reinjection, topical vasoconstrictors, packing, vessel ligation, and possibly even arterial embolization. When bleeding comes from the anterior vessels, it is typically easily controlled with topical vasoconstrictors or light cautery. In the case of a posterior bleed, nasal packing is first attempted, followed by surgical vessel ligation, and then interventional radiology consult for embolization as a last resort. In the author's (CJN) experience of 12 years, this should be an extremely rare event in septoplasty surgery.

In the following hours to days after septoplasty, a hematoma is a surgical emergency in that it can cause a fast-acting pressure necrosis of the septal mucosa as well as the cartilage itself. Presentation

Table 1 Complications of septoplasty	
Early	**Late**
Hematoma	Septal perforation
Excess bleeding	Infection
Infection	Saddle nose deformity
Cerebrospinal fluid leak	Tip ptosis
Pain	Residual deformity or deviation
Reaction to local anesthesia	Internal nasal valve collapse
	Intranasal scarring or adhesions
	Cartilage or mucosal necrosis

would include nasal obstruction, pain, fever, and the presence of an ecchymotic midline nasal mass (**Fig. 12**). Treatment should include prompt drainage of the hematoma, light packing, and oral antibiotics. Major reconstruction of the septum could be required if such an event goes untreated and a perforation results.[9]

Infection of the septum early after a septoplasty with rhinoplasty should be a rare occurrence unless a foreign material is used during the procedure, such as GORE-TEX or similar. Presentation will likely include fever, headache, and nasal discharge with a foul odor. Antibiotic prophylaxis preoperatively should include coverage of gram-positive aerobic bacteria. A septal abscess should be considered an emergency, as inadequate treatment could lead to the devastating complication of cavernous sinus thrombosis.[9] According to Rajan and colleagues,[10] a single preoperative intravenous dose of antibiotics is adequate to prevent postoperative infections.

The presence of a CSF leak should be suspected when the patient presents with complaints of a headache in the postoperative period, especially when a clear nasal discharge is seen. Symptoms can be mild, however, and rhinorrhea may be the only sign. High resection of the perpendicular plate of the ethmoid bone with closed forceps and fracture of the cribriform plate is the most common cause. Treatment initially includes bed rest and antibiotics. If persistent, a neurology consult is indicated and management is beyond the scope of this article.

LATE COMPLICATIONS FROM SEPTOPLASTY

Late complications from septoplasty can range from 1 week to several months postoperatively. The incidence of these potential problems stresses the importance of thorough, routine follow-up examinations until all signs of normal healing have

occurred. Septal perforation is an uncommon but problematic complication of a septoplasty (**Fig. 13**). Causes of septal perforation include mucosal tears (particularly when bilateral and overlapping), untreated or unrecognized septal hematoma, and preoperative use of recreational drugs, particularly intranasal cocaine. Less common causes would include postoperative infection, delayed removal of splints or packing, or overly tight septal mucosal sutures.

Infection after a septoplasty is an extremely uncommon complication in the authors' experience, likely because of the extensive and redundant blood supply to the area of interest. Antibiotics are rarely indicated in the postoperative course but should be prescribed when the patient complains of fever, pain, or purulent, foul-smelling nasal drainage.[9]

Saddle nose deformity and tip ptosis from loss of support should be rare occurrences when conservative principles of resection are followed, as described by Cottle. As described previously, leaving at least 1.5 cm of cartilage in the dorsal and caudal aspects of the septum should nearly eliminate the possibility of nasal collapse.

Internal nasal valve collapse or scarring causing obstruction is typically the result of incisions in this narrow region and also from excess removal of supporting cartilage of the upper and lower lateral cartilages. Intranasal examination will likely show adhesions between the superior aspect of the septum and the lateral nasal wall or turbinate. Repair should include lysis of adhesions and placement of spreader grafts.[9] This problem can be a result of either an "open" or endonasal

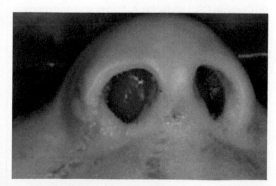

Fig. 12. Nasal septal hematoma.

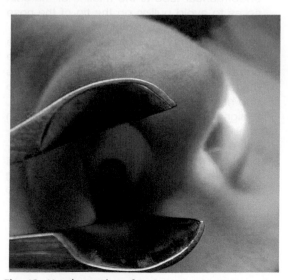

Fig. 13. Nasal septal perforation.

approach. Repair is best accomplished with the placement of spreader grafts between the dorsal septum and upper lateral cartilages.

Residual septal deformity causing obstruction is most common when inadequate repair was done at the time of the initial surgery. The caudal septal cartilage has significant "memory" and will want to return to its native position during the healing period. The use of splints, grafts, scoring, and suturing (or a combination of these) should all contribute to the success of septal cartilage straightening and an improved airway. In the authors' experience, complete release of the soft tissue attachments to the deformed cartilage before remodeling will give the best chance for successful repair in septoplasty surgery.

SEPTOPLASTY PEARLS

1. Be sure that the dissection is in the subperichondrial plane when elevating septal flaps. If there is any bloody tissue over the surface of the cartilage, there may be a layer of perichondrium left. This will help prevent a septal perforation from forming during the healing process.
2. To correct a spur along the floor, a subperiosteal tunnel can be dissected along the floor and connected to the dissection above the junction of the septum and maxillary crest. This will minimize the chance of tearing the mucosal flap along the maxillary crest.
3. Addressing the nasal septum during a cosmetic rhinoplasty is the key to straightening a crooked dorsum as well as improving the nasal airway and/or relieving obstruction.
4. When general anesthesia is used, tape the endotracheal tube to the midline of the chin so as to avoid pulling on the tip of the nose and creating a false midline.
5. After dissecting between the medial crura to approach the septum, the footplates can be sutured to the midline caudal septum. This maneuver will create a more stable nasal tip and help prevent future ptosis.
6. If significant bleeding is noted, the surgeon can first reinject the mucosal flaps with lidocaine with epinephrine and place neurosurgical pledgets, moist with phenylephrine, bilaterally to provide vasoconstriction. During the preparation for surgery, inject into the subperichondrial plane to hydro-dissect the mucosal flaps and aid in their elevation.
7. Avoid beta-blocker medications preoperatively, as the unopposed alpha receptors can lead to flash pulmonary edema.
8. Always preserve dorsal and caudal support with a minimum of 1.5 cm of cartilage in an "L" strut.
9. Even when trimming what seems like unusable small pieces of cartilage or bone, NEVER discard the harvested tissue until the case is completed, as need for additional graft material may arise at any time!
10. Recognize complications early and know how to treat them!
11. The external (open) approach is best for treating the crooked or twisted nasal dorsum.[5]

REFERENCES

1. Brain DJ. Historical background. In: Settipane GA, editor. Nasal polyps: epidemiology, pathogenesis and treatment. Rhode Island: Oceanside Publications; 1997.
2. Stankiewicz JA. Complications in endoscopic intranasal ethmoidectomie. An update. Laryngoscope 1989;99:686–90.
3. Behrbohm H, Tardy M. Essentials of septorhinoplasty. New York: Thieme; 2004.
4. Kim D, Toriumi D. Management of posttraumatic nasal deformities: the crooked nose and the saddle nose. Facial Plast Surg Clin North Am 2004;12:111–32.
5. Toriumi D, Becker D. Rhinoplasty dissection manual. Philadelphia: Lippincott Williams & Wilkins; 1999.
6. Guyuron B. Is packing after septorhinoplasty necessary? A randomized study. Plast Reconstr Surg 1989;84:41–4.
7. Joseph E, Glasgold A. Anatomical considerations in the management of the hanging columella. Arch Facial Plast Surg 2000;2:173–7.
8. Johnson C, Godin M. The tension nose: open structure rhinoplasty approach. Plast Reconstr Surg 1995;95(1):43–51.
9. Cochran CS, Landecker A. Prevention and management of rhinoplasty complications. Plast Reconstr Surg 2008;122(2):60e–7e.
10. Rajan G, Fergie N, Fischer U, et al. Antibiotic prophylaxis in septorhinoplasty? A prospective, randomized study. Plast Reconstr Surg 2005;116: 1995–8.

Grafting in Cosmetic Rhinoplasty

James Koehler, MD, DDS[a,b,*], Landon McLain, MD, DMD[c]

KEYWORDS

- Rhinoplasty • Cosmetic rhinoplasty • Grafting
- Graft techniques

Rhinoplasty has long been regarded as one of the most challenging disciplines in cosmetic surgery. This is because of the elegant combination of form and function inherent to the nose itself. To achieve an esthetically pleasing result to a primary or secondary case, often significant alterations must occur without sacrificing proper physiology and/or the structural integrity of the nasal apparatus. Also, the nose lies directly between the 2 most important features of the face: the eyes and the mouth. A beautiful nose is one that is pleasing to the eye when viewed in isolation, but does not detract from the eyes and mouth, where animation and posture communicate emotion to the observer. An unsatisfactory nose would be one that draws the observer's eye away from the aforementioned features of nonverbal emotion.

Critical to becoming not only an accomplished, but at the very least a competent rhinoplasty surgeon, is a complete understanding of the physiology and anatomy of the nasal apparatus and its supporting structures. This is outside the scope of this article and is already well covered in articles elsewhere in this issue; however, a brief discussion of the anatomic philosophy is prudent for understanding the pearls and pitfalls of grafting in rhinoplasty.

A systematic formula for evaluating the nose is necessary and has been discussed in detail in the literature.[1–4] Perhaps the most common formulation is the one espoused by Johnson and To.[3] Their method focuses on 4 components: the tripod, pedestal, dorsum, and soft tissue envelope. The tripod is composed of the combination of the medial crura to form the medial limb and the lateral crura, which forms the lateral limbs. The pedestal comprises the cartilaginous septum and the anterior nasal spine. The dorsum is made up of both the cartilaginous middle vault (dorsal cartilaginous septum joined with the upper lateral cartilages) and the paired nasal bones adjoining the frontal bone to form the upper vault. The soft tissue envelope is formed by the multiple layers of the skin, subdermis, and nasal vasculature. The manipulation of these parameters allows the rhinoplasty surgeon to manipulate the lower third of the nose to affect rotation, projection, and shape.

In primary rhinoplasty, suboptimal results may occur early or late and are often attributable to weakening of the underlying framework, especially with reductive techniques. This lack of support often leads to buckling of the cartilaginous framework and late deformation after rhinoplasty. This has resulted in more structural grafting during primary and revision procedures and an increasing popularity of the open technique, which offers the advantage of easier visualization and placement of grafts. In the revision nose, it often is overreduction as a whole or differentially without proper structural support that lends to patient dissatisfaction in many cases and motivates the patient to seek correction. These corrections often require reconstitution of the deficient anatomic components. In both cases, an absolute understanding of graft types and techniques is required to tailor the surgical technique to the unique needs of the patient. This article reviews the various graft materials as well as the techniques and indications for their use.

[a] Private Practice, Tulsa Surgical Arts 7322 East 91st Street, Tulsa, OK 74133, USA
[b] Oklahoma State University, 700 North Greenwood Avenue, Tulsa, OK 74106, USA
[c] Private Practice, Carolinas Center for Cosmetic Surgery, 8738 University City Boulevard, Charlotte, NC 28213, USA
* Corresponding author.
E-mail address: james@tulsasurgicalarts.com

Oral Maxillofacial Surg Clin N Am 24 (2012) 59–66
doi:10.1016/j.coms.2011.10.010
1042-3699/12/$ – see front matter © 2012 Elsevier Inc. All rights reserved.

GRAFT MATERIALS

Unfortunately, no ideal graft material exists at this time. Currently, autologous cartilage is the gold standard and many times is readily attainable during septoplasty; however, in revision cases or cases that need additional grafting, the septal cartilage may be a deficient or inadequate donor site. This leads to the problem of creating a separate donor site (conchal bowl or rib) with additional risk and surgical time. Homologous and alloplastic graft materials are indicated at this point and allow the surgeon to add considerable volume to deficient tissues without additional surgery. Injectable grafts (hyaluronic acid or liquid silicone) are occasionally used for minor corrections and asymmetries and can improve outcomes significantly while obviating the need for a second surgery.

AUTOGRAFT

Autogenous grafts are tissues harvested from the patients themselves and vary in tissue types. They are particularly advantageous given their resistance to infection and extrusion and lack of potential disease transmission. The most commonly used autograft in rhinoplasty is septal cartilage (**Fig. 1**A). It is versatile, convenient, and requires little extra effort to obtain grafts with sufficient quantity and quality to suffice in most primary rhinoplasty cases. It can be used for spreader grafts, tip grafts, alar grafting, rim grafts, columellar struts, and small-volume dorsal onlay grafts. Crushed septal cartilage is commonly used to provide volume and soften transition zones, usually at the tip or rhinion. Septal cartilage can be harvested from an endonasal approach or an open approach via either an anterior-superior, dome division technique or from an anterior-inferior approach posterior to the columella as

a hemi-transfixion incision or Killian incision. It is important to leave approximately 1-cm struts anteriorly and dorsally to preserve support for the dorsum and avoid saddle nose deformity (see **Fig. 1**B).

In revision cases, it is common to find inadequate septal cartilage for any necessary grafting. Auricular or conchal bowl cartilage is usually the next most convenient donor site. The primary disadvantage of this donor site is the addition of a second surgical site and potential for complications. Also, conchal bowl cartilage is curved and has elastic memory that makes it less desirable than septal cartilage. This memory usually requires sutured stacking of the graft to counter the contour problems associated with its inherent architecture. Stacking also adds strength and volume to the graft. Most commonly, the conchal bowl is approached from a posterior approach after the ear has been prepped and draped into the surgical field. It can be wise to use the ear opposite of the patient's preferred sleep side, as some post-surgical discomfort is expected. The entirety of the conchal bowl can be harvested, preserving the antihelical fold and the cartilaginous strut from the helical crus. This will preserve auricular architecture postoperatively.

Costochondral grafts are an excellent source of abundant structural graft for large and severe deficits. They have long been used for reconstruction in various parts of the body, including the ear, temporomandibular joint, and the nose.[5–11] They are especially useful in patients requiring revision rhinoplasty or patients who have had septoplasty.

This allows the surgeon to harvest usually more than enough cartilage for even the most deficient and difficult nose.

Commonly the fifth or sixth rib is chosen as the harvest site, as it allows the incision to be hidden in the inframammary crease. The "floater" rib has

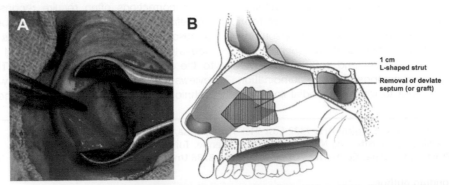

1 cm
L-shaped strut

Removal of deviate
septum (or graft)

Fig. 1. (*A*) Septal cartilage exposed for harvesting graft material for rhinoplasty. (*B*) Preserving a 1-cm strut dorsally and caudally to ensure adequate support for the nose. (*From* Koehler JK, Waite PD. Basic principles of rhinoplasty. In: Miloro M, editor. Oral and maxillofacial surgery. Hamilton: BC Decker; 2004; with permission.)

been espoused by some as more ideal because of presumed resistance to warping.[12] It is the authors' preference to use the right side to avoid confusing any potential postoperative pain with that of cardiac origin. The incision is typically 4 to 5 cm in length and lies within the inframammary fold (which should be marked with the patient in the seated or standing position). Dissection proceeds quickly down through the skin, subcutaneous tissues, rectus fascia, and muscle. The perichondrium is divided carefully and subperichondreal dissection proceeds carefully around the circumference of the rib. Cutting the lateral aspect of the rib and careful elevation of the perichondrium away from its ventral surface will reduce the risk of pleural violation. It is prudent to always check for pneumothorax with saline and Valsalva maneuvers before layered closure. The central core of the rib is the most beneficial component, as the eccentric portions are more prone to warping (**Fig. 2**).[13] Some surgeons even advocate use of a steel pin or K-wire to promote fixation and prevent late warping.[14]

Autogenous bone grafts are useful in reconstruction of the upper third of the nasal vault. Calvarial, iliac crest, and rib are the most common sources. Calvarial bone is membranous in origin and more resistant to resorption than iliac crest and has less donor site morbidity.[15] Rib cartilage is preferred versus rib bone grafts. Although these materials have a long history of use in reconstructive rhinoplasty, they are less common to cosmetic rhinoplasty given the donor site risks, invasiveness of harvesting, and potential for contour irregularities.

ALLOGRAFT

Allografts are grafts derived from human cadavers. Bone allografts are common to orthopedics, spinal surgery, and oral surgery. In cosmetic rhinoplasty, the most common alloplastic graft is acellular dermal matrix. This is sterilized dermis taken from prescreened cadaveric donors that comes in a variety of thicknesses and sizes. Given the significant early resorption, these materials are best used for graft camouflage under a thin soft tissue envelope, particularly in the rhinion area.

ALLOPLAST

Alloplastic grafts are synthetic grafts of various materials ranging from silicone to polytetrafluoroethylene (PTFE) to polydiaxone (PDS). These materials are usually reserved for the deficient nasal dorsum. There appears to be an upswing in the use of these materials in recent years given their availability, ease of use, and tolerance by the host tissues. Any implant material can be successful given proper integration and conformation. Each material does have specific advantages and disadvantages, however. Porous implants (ie, porous polyethylene) influence the risk of fibrous ingrowth and infection (**Fig. 3**). This can be a significant advantage in stabilizing the implant, but can pose a significant problem if removal or repositioning is required. As there is no distinct fibrous capsule, the removal can be traumatic for the adjacent tissues, which are oftentimes composed of muscle and nerve. There is also a high potential for graft fragmentation given the difficulty of removal. This can result in leaving small graft particles behind.

Solid silicone implants, on the other hand, form a distinct fibrous capsule without tissue ingrowth. This allows easier removal if needed, but increases the risk of extrusion. It is the authors' preference to fixate silicone implants whenever feasible to minimize the risk of malpositioning or extrusion. This is usually achieved via percutaneous miniscrew fixation or suturing techniques. Another advantage to solid silicone is the flexible nature of the graft. This allows smaller access for placement and increased forgiveness if the implant does not lay in absolute intimacy on the underneath dorsum (**Fig. 4**).

Of particular note when discussing silicone is the use of liquid silicone in rhinoplasty (**Fig. 5**).

A

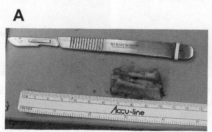

B

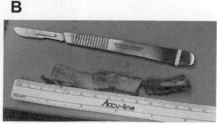

Fig. 2. (*A*) A 4-cm section of costal cartilage that has been sectioned for nasal reconstruction. The most suitable piece is the middle one because it will be the least prone to warping and distortion. (*B*) When extensive grafting is required, the rib provides an abundant source for structural support for the nose.

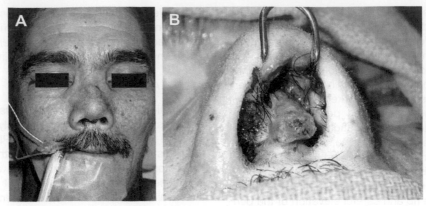

Fig. 3. (A) Patient at surgery to remove an infected alloplastic dorsal graft that had been in place for 5 years. Patient was a heavy smoker. (B) No incision was made, as the graft had begun extruding through the columella. The material appeared to be porous, high-density polyethylene.

Liquid silicone has both been revered and condemned as a filler over the years. In the past, unscrupulous practitioners have used industrial-grade (instead of medical-grade) silicone to add volume to various parts of the body. The impurities and massive volumes used led to a host of well-documented problems.[16,17] On the other hand, proper use of medical-grade liquid silicone

(approved by the Food and Drug Administration for ophthalmic use) has a number of advantages, including ease of use, painless injection, natural feel, minimal side effects, and permanence. This allows the rhinoplasty surgeon to use a safe, permanent material to camouflage graft contours, augment mildly overreduced areas (commonly the supratip break), and enhance tip-defining points

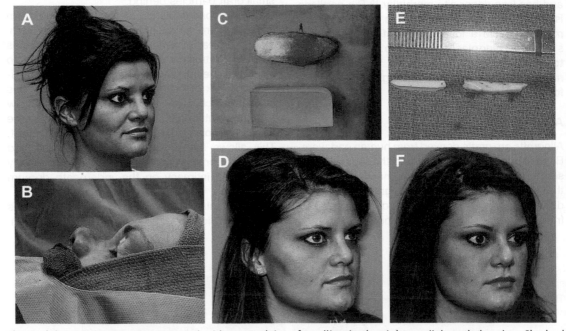

Fig. 4. (A) A young woman presented with a complaint of swelling in the right medial canthal region. She had previous nasal surgery done with grafting but was unsure what material was used. (B) Patient's nasal dorsum after graft was removed. Significant saddle nose deformity was present. (C) Infected expanded PTFE (ePTFE) graft was removed and placed next to a block of silicone that was carved as a temporary graft to be used as a spacer after debridement of the nose. (D) Three months after removal of the ePTFE and placement of carved silicone graft. (E) Silicone graft on left with carved rib cartilage on right in preparation for placement. (F) Three months after placement of rib graft.

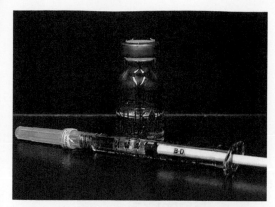

Fig. 5. Liquid silicone of 1000 centistokes can be cautiously used to fill small soft tissue defects after rhinoplasty. Use of this is off label and patients should be informed of this along with potential risks.

and oftentimes eliminate the need for a revision surgery in an unsatisfied patient. The caveat is the strict avoidance of overcorrection. The patient must be made aware that treatment with liquid silicone requires multiple injections and is a stepwise sculpting process.

SPECIFIC GRAFT TECHNIQUES

The literature is replete with graft techniques for cosmetic rhinoplasty. Many are just variations on a theme and their sheer volume when accounted for individually can be exhausting and confusing. It is often best to categorize the graft techniques according to anatomic zones (upper vault, middle vault, and lower vault). This article focuses on the most common techniques specific to the aforementioned zones. Invariably, the discussion of grafting leads to the controversy of which approach to use, either open versus endonasal. That argument is beyond the scope of this text, suffice to say that many of these grafting techniques can be used with either approach.

Advocates of the endonasal approach extol the absence of a collumellar scar and decreased postoperative tip edema (although this has never been scientifically proven). In our experience, the open approach allows better visualization for proper diagnosis, treatment, and easier grafting. The columellar scar is typically inconspicuous if the tissues are handled gently and the closure is precise. Prolonged tip edema has not been noticeably different with either approach in our experience. This has resulted in our using the open approach for most cases, withholding the endonasal approach for simple dorsal reduction cases that require minimal if any tip modification.

Upper Vault

The upper vault is composed of the paired nasal bones and their cartilaginous junction as well as the nasal process of the frontal bone. This comprises the radix and bony dorsum primarily.

Deficiency of the radix is commonly overlooked and can lead to improper or overreduction of the dorsum, which can result in significant deformity for the patient. Grafts to the radix primarily are performed to augment the nasofrontal angle. This essentially moves the radix cephalad and gives the appearance of added nasal length.

Given the thicker soft tissue envelope in this region, contour irregularity and asymmetry is less common with this graft. Most surgeons use autologous cartilage or bone for this procedure.

The dorsal onlay graft is perhaps the most common indication for alloplastic graft materials. PTFE and solid silicone are the usual formats; however, autologous rib cartilage or bone is frequently used also (see **Fig. 4**). This graft typically repairs acquired nasal deformities, such as saddle nose, excessive reduction from prior rhinoplasty, or deformity after trauma. Dorsal grafting is often indicated in ethnic rhinoplasty as well, where lack of length and dorsal projection is common. This is usually combined with significant augmentation of the underlying nasal skeleton. Depending on graft type, suture or miniscrew fixation may be used. Precise pocket development combined with fixation greatly decreases the risk of mobility or migration. We have had great success with both solid silicone and sculpted costochondral cartilage in this setting (see **Fig. 4**).

Lateral Nasal Wall

Dorsal sidewall grafts are rarely used but are useful when treating focal depressions along the dorsal sidewall, typically resultant from lateral osteotomies. These are typically crushed cartilage but the increasing use of filler treatment has abated the need for these grafts.

Middle Vault

The upper lateral cartilages and cartilaginous septum comprise the framework of the middle vault and house the internal nasal valve. The internal nasal valve is formed by the aforementioned cartilaginous framework and the respective angle between them. Because this is the point of greatest resistance to airflow through the upper airway, loss of patency, either partial or total, here can lead to significant obstruction. This can be corrected with the use of spreader grafts (**Fig. 6**).

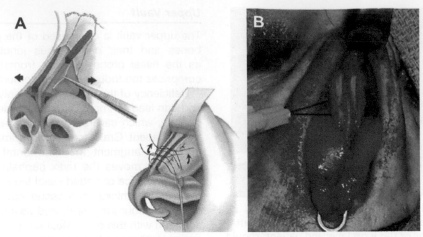

Fig. 6. (*A*) Schematic for the placement of spreader grafts to prevent internal nasal valve collapse (*From* Dolan R. Nasal valve and nasal alar dysfunction. In: GR Holt, editor. Facial Plastic Surgery Clinics of North America 2000;8(4):447–64; with permission.). (*B*) Intraoperative picture of spreader grafts temporarily being stabilized with 27 gauge needles.

The primary function of spreader grafts is to increase the angle between the dorsal septum and the upper lateral cartilages and prevent or correct internal nasal valve collapse and/or correct open roof deformity. These can be preemptively placed in patients at risk for internal valve collapse after rhinoplasty, such as revision cases or in patients with short nasal bones. Typically, these grafts are 3 to 5 mm in thickness and extend from a point just cephalic to the anterior septal angle to the osseocartilaginous junction. Spreader grafts may also be extended beyond the anterior septal angle to join and stabilize a columellar strut (**Fig. 7**). Septal and rib cartilage are the most common donor sites.

Rhinion onlay grafts are useful to camouflage abrupt transitions from the paired nasal bones to the upper lateral cartilages. Given the transition from one tissue type to another (bone to cartilage or vice versa) combined with the thinness of the soft tissue envelope, the rhinion is prone to contour irregularity and palpable deformities. Crushed cartilage as well as acellular dermal matrix have served well in this situation. These, along with, less commonly, perichondrium or temporalis fascia, are useful tools when performing rhinoplasty in thin-skinned patients who are predisposed to having visible contour irregularities postoperatively.

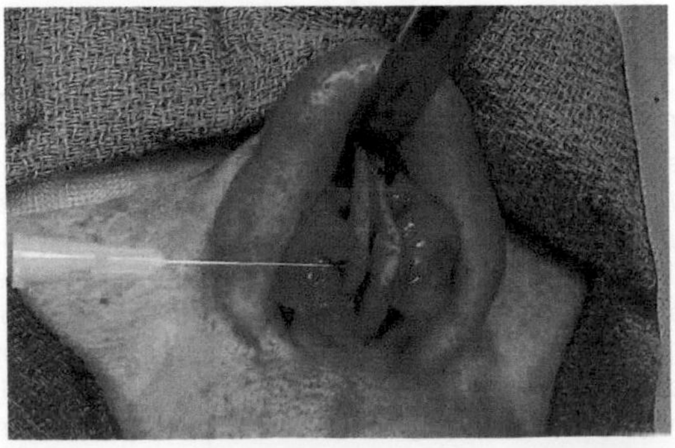

Lower Vault

Grafting in the lower vault and tip of the nose is oftentimes the most complex, given the intricate anatomy and the preponderance of focus by both the patient and the observer in this area. This anatomic zone of the nose also has the most diversity in grafting techniques. Columellar strut grafts are one of the most common techniques to provide structural support to the nasal tip as well as provide increased projection while affecting tip rotation (**Fig. 8**). This graft can be placed through either an endonasal or traditional open technique as well as via a vertical skin incision through the columella between the medial crura. There is some controversy regarding the ideal length for the strut. Many advocate leaving the caudal portion short of the nasal spine to prevent clicking or lateral displacement over time. Others prefer to engage the anterior nasal spine with a v-notch in the end of the strut. In our experience, there is no inherent advantage to engaging the anterior nasal spine, as a well-fashioned columellar strut placed short of the premaxilla seems to provide more than enough support to the nasal tip while avoiding clicking or

Fig. 7. Extended spreader grafts made of rib cartilage connected to a columellar strut graft.

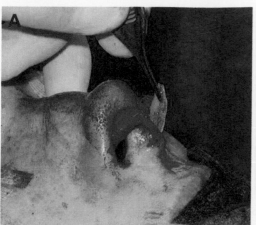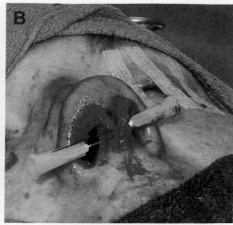

Fig. 8. (*A*) Septal cartilage being placed between the medial crura for a columellar strut. (*B*) Temporary stabilization of the columellar strut with 27-gauge needles before suture fixation with 5-0 prolene suture.

deformity with facial animation. It is important not to overextend the strut unless advancing the lower lateral crura to increase tip projection, otherwise a "unidome" deformity may occur.

Tip grafts come in many shapes and sizes. The prevailing theme is to increase tip projection but they can also add definition to the tip or even soften the bifid or cleft tip. They are typically derived from autologous sources, such as the conchal bowl, septum, or from cephalic trimming, and can be stacked to increase projection. The edges should be beveled to smooth transition points. This can be done with a scalpel or a diamond bur per the surgeon's preference. If placed below the domes they can also increase the infratip lobule definition. One benefit for the open technique is the ability to accurately secure these grafts with fine sutures. It is desirable to bury knots and use smaller caliber suture whenever possible to avoid palpability or extrusion. The most common tip grafts are shield grafts or Sheen grafts, cap grafts, and anchor grafts. Shield grafts are positioned over the medial crura and extend up to or just beyond the domes. These grafts add volume to the infratip lobule, increase tip projection, and may be modified to promote tip-defining points. They are best reserved for patients with a normal to thick soft tissue envelope, as they can be conspicuous in thin-skinned patients. Cap grafts typically are secured over the domes and are useful to diminish clefting of the nasal tip and add some volume to the tip. Anchor grafts are less commonly used than the aforementioned techniques but can help in correcting the pinched nasal tip with inadequate infratip volume.

Alar grafts are useful in correction and/or prophylaxis of external nasal valve collapse. The external nasal valve is primarily composed of the lower lateral cartilages and their respective soft tissue covering. Collapse of this aperture can lead to altered nasal airflow and even obstruction. This has many etiologies ranging from inherent weakness of the lower lateral cartilages, overresection and iatrogenic weakening of the cartilages, to overprojection of the tip resulting in slitlike nares.[18] Although much focus has been on internal nasal valve dynamics, it is our opinion that at least equal attention must be paid to the external nasal valve.

Alar batten grafts are applied external to the lower lateral cartilages and centered over the region of maximal collapse or weakness. They can be placed either slightly cephalic to the superior crural margin to improve internal nasal valve function or slightly caudal to the inferior margin to correct mild alar rim retraction. Septal and auricular cartilage are most common and can be attached to PDS mesh to increase stability of the graft material (**Fig. 9**). Alar rim grafts are placed abutting the inferior margin of the lower lateral crura and are used to correct alar retraction. Severe cases may warrant composite grafts composed of skin, perichondrium, and cartilage. These may be harvested from the cavum cymba, cavum concha, or auricular root. The donor site is then closed with a full-thickness skin graft from the post auricular region. Alar strut grafts are a preferable option for very thin-skinned patients with mild to moderate alar collapse in whom batten grafts may provide an unesthetic result. These grafts are placed on the ventral

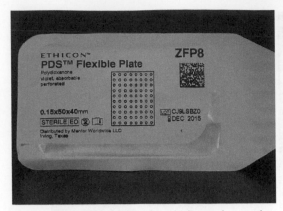

Fig. 9. PDS resorbable mesh, which can be used to stabilize cartilage grafts in rhinoplasty.

surface of the lateral crura between the cartilage and the nasal mucosa. These are technically more challenging to place versus alar batten grafts and provide less structural support.

Other

Premaxillary grafting is a useful adjunct to augment the retrusive maxilla. Many of these patients require Lefort advancement ideally, but may be unwilling to undergo the extended treatment time typically required. The augmented premaxilla can improve nasolabial conformation and when combined with columellar plumping grafts can improve the retracted columella and acute nasolabial angle, giving the appearance f superior tip rotation. This is a frequent requirement in patients with cleft and Asian patients, who commonly display maxillary hypoplasia.

SUMMARY

As rhinoplasty techniques continue to evolve toward structural support and away from purely reductive techniques, the need for sophisticated grafting options will escalate to augment or replace critical support mechanisms of the nose. This will result in not only improved esthetic outcomes but functional results as well. Obviously, the goal is to provide the patient with the most elegant nose possible given their preoperative conformation while providing a result that will stand the test of time. We have found that well-planned and executed adjunctive grafting techniques can deliver lasting results with preservation of function as well as cosmesis.

REFERENCES

1. Swartout B, Toriumi DM. Rhinoplasty. Curr Opin Oto-laryngol Head Neck Surg 2001;15:219–27.

2. Kim DW, Toriumi DM. Nasal analysis for secondary rhinoplasty. Facial Plast Surg Clin North Am 2003; 11:399–419.

3. Johnson CM, Wyatt CT. The tripod-pedestal concept, vol 1. A case approach to open structure rhinoplasty. Michigan: Elsevier-Saunders; 2005. p. 9–20.

4. Whitaker EG, Johnson CM Jr. The evolution of open structure rhinoplasty. Arch Facial Plast Surg 2003; 5(4):291–300.

5. Tasanen AK, Nordling L. Central giant cell lesion in the mandibular condyle. Report of a case. Oral Surg Oral Med Oral Pathol 1978;45(4):532–9.

6. Figueroa AA, Ganz BJ, Pruzansky S. Long-term follow-up of a mandibular costochondral graft. Oral Surg Oral Med Oral Pathol 1984;58(3):257–68.

7. Brent B. Ear reconstruction with an expansile frame-work of autogenous rib cartilage. Plast Reconstr Surg 1974;53(6):619–28.

8. Avelar J. A new technique for reconstruction of the auricle in acquired deformities. Ann Plast Surg 1987;18(5):454–64.

9. Lazaro CC, Maria TG. Use of cartilaginous auto-grafts in nasal surgery: 8 years of experience. Plast Reconstr Surg 1999;103:1003–14.

10. Judith MG, Thomas P, Chad AP, et al. Long-term outcome of autogenous rib graft nasal reconstruc-tion. Plast Reconstr Surg 2001;108:1895–907.

11. Laurence AC, Hilton B, Alex C. The versatile costal osteochondral graft in nasal reconstruction. Br J Plast Surg 1980;33:179–84.

12. Christophel JJ, Hilger PA. Osseocartilaginous rib graft in rhinoplasty: a stable, predictable technique for major dorsal reconstruction. Arch facial Plast Surg 2011;13(2):78–83.

13. Immerman S, White M, Constanides M. Cartilage grafting in nasal reconstruction. Facial Plast Surg Clin North Am 2011;19(1):175–82.

14. Kim KK, Zhao L, Belafsky P, et al. Technical note: "look-ahead" navigation method for K-wire fixation in rhinoplasty. Oral Surg Oral Med Oral Pathol Oral Radiol Endod 2008;105(2):168–72.

15. Frodel JL Jr, Marentette LJ, Weinstein GS. Calvarial bone graft harvest. Techniques, considerations, and morbidity. Arch Otolaryngol Head Neck Surg 1993;119(1):17–23.

16. Hage JJ, Kanhai RC, Oen AL, et al. The devastating outcome of massive subcutaneous injection of highly viscous fluids in male-to-female transsexuals. Plast Reconstr Surg 2001;107(3):734–41.

17. Klein AW, Elson LE. The history of substances for soft tissue augmentation. Dermatol Surg 2000; 26(12):1096–105.

18. Constantian MB. The incompetent external nasal valve: pathophysiology and treatment in primary and secondary rhinoplasty. Plast Reconstr Surg 1994;93(5):919–31.

Nasal Tip Modifications

Mary L. Schinkel, DO[a],*, L. Mike Nayak, MD[b,c]

KEYWORDS

- Nasal tip • Tip modifications • Tip rhinoplasty • Rhinoplasty
- Suture techniques

The nasal tip is to the rhinoplasty what the nose is to the face, the centerpiece. The entire rhinoplasty hinges on the creation of a strong, symmetric, defined and well-projected nasal tip. Only when these goals are achieved can there be harmony of the nasal anatomy.[1] Over the past several decades, the nasal tip supporting mechanisms have been understood and described in detail. Modern rhinoplasty techniques use this new understanding to preserve and control tip support, while enhancing nasal esthetics.[1,2] The techniques accomplishing these goals have been at the heart of a paradigm shift in aesthetic rhinoplasty over this time frame.[2]

The main objectives in a primary rhinoplasty are controlling shape, definition, rotation and projection of the nasal tip while preserving its integrity.[3] The anatomic structures, which are the focus of these goals, are the lower lateral cartilages and their relationships with the surrounding nasal anatomy (**Figs. 1** and **2**).

The lower lateral cartilages provide tip support through the formation of a functional tripod described in 1969.[4] This idea, known as the Anderson tripod concept, proposed a new understanding of tip dynamics. It consists of the combined medial crura as one leg and each of the lateral crura as the other legs of this tripod. This theory has been the foundation for tip projection, support and rotation for 40 years.[5] The supportive tripod exists to counteract the majority of the inherent external forces on the nose, which are oriented in a posterocaudal direction.[6]

Johnson and Toriumi[7] decried the disruptive techniques performed during rhinoplasty over 20 years ago. They espoused a need to maintain tip support, to prevent the collapse of the lower lateral cartilages due to the contractile forces of long-term healing. Their solution was the preservation of the ligamentous attachments to the nasal tip, which, in turn, maintained the integrity of the tip and the internal nasal valve.[7] These ligamentous attachments are part of the mechanisms responsible for nasal tip support. These supportive mechanisms of the nasal tip were described in 1969 by Anderson[4] and in 1971 by Janeke and Wright.[8] These supports were further illustrated by Tardy in the late 1990s[9] and quantitatively evaluated by Beatty and colleagues 5 years later.[10] Anderson detailed 7 mechanisms[4] whereas Janeke and Wright described 4 major tip supporting structures.[8] These were later modified to 3 major and 6 minor tip supporting mechanisms (**Table 1**).[1,9] The major mechanisms supporting the nasal tip consist of the medial and lateral crura their attachments to the quadrangular cartilage and the upper lateral cartilages.[1,9] Other more minor tip support mechanisms include the membranous and dorsal cartilaginous septum, nasal spine, interdomal ligaments, alar side walls, and attachment of the soft tissue of the nose to the cartilages.[1,9] Some argue for including the interdomal ligament as a major tip supporting mechanism.[8,10,11] Understanding and respecting the interrelationship of these mechanisms is the key to a successful tip modification.[9] In primary rhinoplasty, dividing the ligamentous

The authors have nothing to disclose.

[a] Department of Medical Education, Des Peres Hospital, 2345 Doughterty Ferry Road, St Louis, MO 63122, USA
[b] Nayak Plastic Surgery and Skin Enhancement Center, 607 South Lindbergh Boulevard, St Louis, MO 63131, USA
[c] Department of Otolaryngology–Head and Neck Surgery, Saint Louis University, St Louis, MO, USA
* Corresponding author.
E-mail address: mlschinkel@yahoo.com

Oral Maxillofacial Surg Clin N Am 24 (2012) 67–74
doi:10.1016/j.coms.2011.10.004

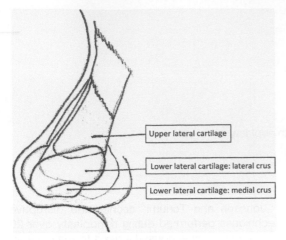

Fig. 1. Nasal cartilages: lateral view.

attachments between the lateral crura results in a 25% decrease in tip support. The suture reconstruction of these ligaments demonstrates a 35% improvement in tip support above the original baseline. Addition of a columellar strut to the ligamentous reconstruction creates a 44% increased tip support.[10] This system of restoring through sutures and grafting the support lost during the initial step in rhinoplasty is commonly known as the deproject/reproject sequence.

The evolution of the rhinoplasty surgery is a shift from cartilage resection and disruption of tip supports, to one of cartilage modification and preservation of these mechanisms. The techniques have changed from resection, scoring and morselizing, to preservation, supporting and defining, with the application of suture techniques.[2] Now the suture has largely replaced the knife in the realm of tip modification. Suturing techniques provide nondestructive and reversible methods to reposition and restructure the nasal tip. A major critique of these procedures has been the potential for extrusion of the sutures. In one study of 233 rhinoplasty surgeries, only 2 cases of suture exposure occurred necessitating

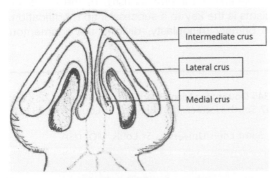

Fig. 2. Lower lateral cartilages: base view.

removal and no deformity resulted from the loss of the suture.[3] The goals of conservation, strengthening and refinement of the lower lateral cartilages and their relationships with the surrounding nasal anatomy are now better realized than ever before.

Aesthetic rhinoplasty remains the most challenging and elegant procedure in the realm of plastic surgery.[1] Every nose presents its own unique obstacles and navigating them requires a systematic approach. In 1994, Tebbetts[3] presented a systematic approach of 4 stages for nasal tip shaping and positioning. Stage 1 detailed soft tissue elevation and cephalic trim. Stage 2 was medial crura unification and dome projection. Stage 3 described lateral crura and dome shaping with suture techniques. Then stage 4 was tip positioning for symmetric projection and rotation. The key techniques, including tip control and projection, were achieved through the use of reversible suture methods. These methods were performed in an incremental fashion without visible grafts.[3] All 4 of these stages culminated in the achievement of the ultimate goal, the "unified, symmetric tip complex."[3]

The steps presented here are a modification of Tebbetts' 4 stages for a systematic approach to the nasal tip. There is certainly no one method to follow for every rhinoplasty. No two procedures are ever identical, although having a basic guide to follow assists in a successful outcome. Always remembering the objectives of conservation, strengthening and refinement is the key to a successful rhinoplasty.[1–8] The purpose of this article are to detail a systematic approach to the nasal tip and propose a basic algorithm for its modifications.

TEN STEPS IN A SYSTEMATIC APPROACH TO NASAL TIP MODIFICATION
Step 1: Surgical Approach

The surgical incisions to the nasal tip include marginal, transfixion, intercartilaginous, and open (transcolumellar). The 3 former incisions are subdivided into delivery and nondelivery methods. These were evaluated for their quantitative effects on tip support.[10] The marginal and transfixion incisions were found to be nondestructive. The intercartilaginous incision divides the intercrural ligament and separates the upper and lower cartilage attachments. This results in a reduction of tip support by 25% and up to 35% with delivery of the lower lateral cartilages.[10] The open approach was better at preserving tip support than the closed approaches in this study, which emphasized the importance of the intercrural ligament in supporting the nasal tip.[10] Even within the realm of the

Table 1 Supporting mechanisms to the nasal tip		
Anderson,[4] 1969	**Janeke and Wright,[8] 1971**	**Tardy,[9] 1997**

Lateral crural scroll ligaments
Medial crural ligaments
Caudal upper lateral cartilages
Membranous septum
Medial crura
Premaxillary fat pad
Lateral crura
	Ligaments of upper and lower
	  lateral cartilages
	Sesamoid complex from
	  lateral crura
	Lower lateral cartilage domal
	  ligaments
	Medial crura attachments to
	  caudal septum
		Major
		  Medial and lateral crura
		  Medial crural and caudal
		    septum ligaments
		  Upper and lower lateral
		    cartilage ligaments
		Minor
		  Cartilaginous septum
		  Interdomal ligaments
		  Membranous septum
		  Nasal spine
		  Skin and soft tissue
		  Alar side walls

open approach, various midcolumellar incisions exist among surgeons. Incision types include the sharp angled V, inverted V, gull wing, and inverted gull wing (**Fig. 3**).[1] The random pattern of these incisions, regardless of the type, presents a minimal scar in this area.

Tip modifications are the most demanding and most challenging part of rhinoplasty; many surgeons advocate performing them first, then performing dorsal work to match the new tip.[1,11] Other surgeons recommend performing tip procedures after intranasal work and osteotomies to prevent disruption of the new tip structure.[3] There is no guideline for which must be done first. Alteration of the bony nasal dorsum and upper lateral

cartilages would inherently change the dynamic forces on the nasal tip, but a stabilized nasal tip would have the capacity to resist these forces.[3,11]

Step 2: Soft Tissue Elevation

The open or external approach to the nasal septum is the most traumatic to the nasal tip.[12] The resulting trauma is minimized if elevation is performed carefully, under the full thickness of the soft tissue envelope and without disrupting the nasal cartilaginous elements (**Fig. 4**). If these elements and the perichondrium are maintained, there is a reduction in both bleeding and scarring.[3] Also of great importance is preserving any soft

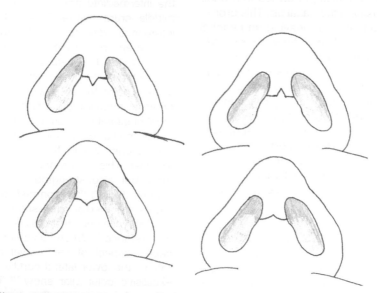

Fig. 3. Midcolumellar incisions: V, upper left; inverted V, upper right; gull wing, lower left; and inverted gull wing, lower right.

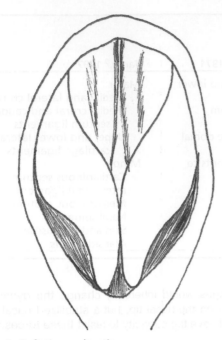

Fig. 4. Soft tissue elevation.

tissue fat during this dissection to prevent thinning and atrophy deformities in the long term. Symmetry is the key to elevating the soft tissue.[3]

Step 3: Cephalic Lateral Cartilage Trim

Symmetry is also crucial to creating the lateral crural rim strips. Resection of the cephalic lateral cartilage should include precise measurements to preserve or create symmetry. This also helps to minimize dead space and the associated fibrosis. The cephalic trim is performed to reduce the bulk and bulbosity of the nasal tip. This procedure should be conservative, leaving an intact 6 mm to 10 mm complete lateral crura strip **(Fig. 5)**.[1,8] The advantage to a 6-mm complete strip is the ease of suture manipulation, while minimizing the risk of alar retraction or collapse.[3,13–15] If reducing the bulky nasal tip does violate the upper lateral cartilage attachments and the sesamoid complex laterally, the remaining mechanism crucial to preserving nasal tip support is the caudal septum connection to the medial crura.[3,8,13,14] Structural grafts, such as columellar struts, shield grafts, or cap grafts, can also replace or reinforce inadequate tip support.[1,3,12]

Step 4: Medial Crura Suture

Understanding the 3-D characteristics of the lower lateral crura is invaluable to mastering the dynamics of suture techniques. A tapered needle is ideal to prevent tearing of the cartilages and the knots should always be positioned medially,

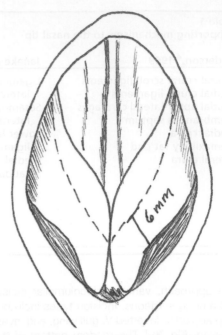

Fig. 5. Cephalic lateral cartilage trim leaving 6-mm complete strip.

between the domes.[3] A 4-0 or 5-0 nylon, prolene, or polydioxanone (PDS) suture on an SH needle is ideal. If with cutting needle is performed, a PS-2 is favored because its shallow curve makes violating the vestibular mucosa less likely.[13,16]

Controlling the shape and position of the medial crura requires establishing the projection symmetry of the dome, shaping and then stabilizing with a 5-0 monofilament. The suture fixation at the cephalic aspect of the medial crura, where the intermediate crura diverge, is known as the middle crura suture. This suture reduces the interdomal distance while increasing lobule volume and protrusion. This suture serves to not only stabilize the medical crura, but also create symmetric dome projection and provide the initial fixation point for all other sutures. This fixation prevents medial crura disruption with the placement of lateral crura sutures **(Fig. 6)**.[3,16,17]

The medial crura suture, when placed at the middle one-third of the crura, brings the crura together. This suture not only narrows the columella but also strengthens it while adding tip support **(Fig. 7)**.[16] In contrast to the middle crura suture, the medial crura suture augments lobule volume while only minimally reducing the interdomal distance.[16] When this suture is placed at the caudal aspect of the medial crura, it caudally rotates the lower lateral cartilages, which benefit excessive columellar show.[16] The medial crura suture also known as flare control suture, these acts to control the amount of crural flare, alter the

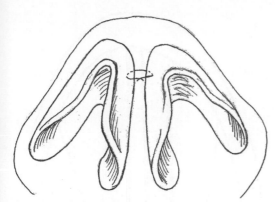

Fig. 6. Middle crura suture at junction of medial crura and intermediate crura.

profile of the columella, resolve asymmetries, and provide for intercrural strut stabilization.[3] These sutures must be at least 2 mm to 3 mm above the caudal border of the medial crura to maintain the normal crural flare. The medial crura unification achieves several objectives: "it shapes and positions the medial crura, it sets basic dome projection symmetry, and it establishes force-termination points to prevent lateral crural and dome transmitted suture forces from displacing or distorting medial crural relationships."[16]

Step 5: Columellar Strut

Next, a columellar strut may be placed at this time. Optimal material for the strut is septal cartilage.[3] It is a multiple function tool in rhinoplasty surgery, with a variety of indications. The columellar strut may increase or decrease tip projection, control the medial crura shape and profile and regulate the columellar-lobular angle. The strut functions to enhance or reduce columellar show, control the nasal length and improve medial crura asymmetries or deformities.[3] If the strut is designed to shape the medial crura, a width of 3 mm to 4

mm and length of 12 mm to 15 mm is sufficient. The width may be increased to correct columellar retraction, serving as a combination caudal septal extension graft and columellar strut. If tip projection greater than 3 mm is required, the strut may be lengthened and placed in contact with the maxillary crest.[3] The strut is always suture fixated into position between the medial crura to prevent malposition, and the ends overlapped to avoid protrusion (**Fig. 8**).[3]

Step 6: Lateral Crural Modifications

At this point the cephalic trim of the lower lateral cartilages has been performed, resulting in at least a 6-mm lateral crural strip, which is stable and may be further modified with a mattress suture.[14] Controlling curvature of the lateral crural to narrow the broad or bulbous tip is the objective. Horizontal mattress sutures have a widely varied usefulness in the correction of convexities and concavities of the nasal tip. These sutures have proved repeatedly to augment the strength of the resulting cartilage, whereas scoring results only in weakening it. These suture techniques are further used in correcting everything from a bulbous tip, to internal and external nasal valve collapse, to straightening curved cartilage grafts and septal struts. The lateral crura suture is a horizontal mattress placed through each of the lateral crura at the middle two-thirds, spanning the caudal nasal septum (**Fig. 9**). This technique results in narrowing the interdomal distance and elongating the nose. Its

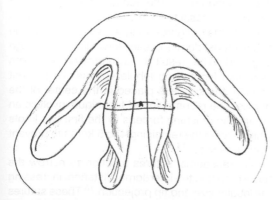

Fig. 7. Medial crura suture at middle one-third of medial crura.

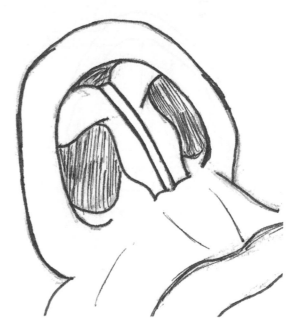

Fig. 8. Columellar strut in position between the medial crura.

purpose is also its greatest complication; excessive tip narrowing is the primary difficulty with this suture, causing nasal obstruction.[11]

The lateral crura convexity control suture is another example of a horizontal mattress suture technique. As its name suggests, this suture's purpose is to straighten the lateral crus by decreasing their convexity. The lateral crus average thickness is 0.5 mm and requires the horizontal mattress to be 6-mm to 8-mm wide for maximal correction of convexity without buckling (**Fig. 10**). For the thicker cartilage of 1.5 mm, a suture spacing of 8 mm to 10 mm is recommended.[13] Care is taken to begin the suture on the caudal aspect; this results in a caudal knot to prevent the possibility of a palpable cephalic knot. Also noted is the lateral movement of the posterior aspect of the lateral crus. These sutures have replaced the scoring technique because the sutures increase lateral crura stiffness by 35% over baseline, whereas scoring decreased stiffness by 48%.[13] Sutures are also inherently reversible as opposed to scoring. If the remaining lateral crura are not long or wide enough for suture placement, a Gunter-type strut may be attached to the vestibular side to improve the convexity.[14] The lateral crura convexity control suture narrows the external nasal valve and may cause a change in nasal function. Excessive tightening must be avoided to prevent further narrowing and compromise of the external valve.[16]

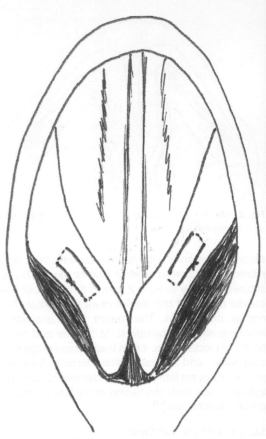

Fig. 10. Lateral crura convexity control suture, 6 mm to 8 mm wide in the 0.5-mm thickness cartilage.

Step 7: Dome Refinement

Shaping the nasal dome is another area of the rhinoplasty that has changed dramatically with the shift in techniques in recent years. The destructive nature of scoring, morselization, or resection increased the risks of buckling, collapse, or contour irregularities. Now the suture techniques augment the strength and integrity of the resulting tip.[3,11] The domal sutures refine and stabilize the nasal tip.[17] The interdomal suture places a simple or figure-of-eight fashion through the anterior most domes of each lower lateral cartilage (**Fig. 11**). The result is a narrowed tip, with increased length and lobule volume. To prevent rotation, the suture is placed in the center of the domes. The recommended technique involves an atraumatic grasping forceps to the first two knots while placing the remaining 4 to 5 knots to prevent overtightening.[3,17]

The transdomal sutures function to narrow the tip by reducing the interdomal distance, increasing the lobular size and tip projection.[16] These sutures are placed through each domal arch in a horizontal mattress fashion, taking care not to penetrate the

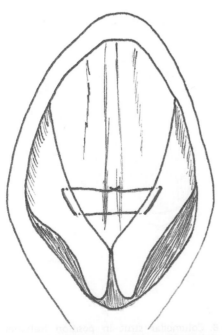

Fig. 9. Lateral crura suture at the middle two-thirds.

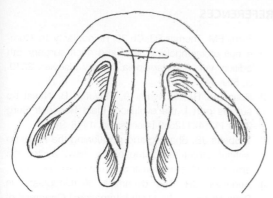

Fig. 11. Interdomal suture.

vestibular lining to prevent suture exposure (**Fig. 12**). The interdomal suture provides greater domal approximation than the transdomal suture.[16] Transdomal sutures may cause medial or superior displacement of the lateral crura, requiring strut grafts or alar rim grafts, respectively.

Step 8: Tip Projection

Many of the tip suture techniques, including the transdomal, intercrural and medial crural sutures, increase the support and projection of the nasal tip. There are also a multitude of grafts to enhance the tip, including infratip lobule, onlay tip, plumping and columellar grafts.[1] Reduction of tip projection has proved more difficult and previously relied on interrupted strip techniques, which were complicated by the potential for healing asymmetry and loss of tip support.[1]

As an alternative, the medial crural-septal suture is used to control nasal tip projection in either direction. Increased tip projection is achieved when the suture is placed through the medial crura footplates, or the posterior crura and the caudal septum. This suture widens the interdomal distance if a medial crura suture was not

previously placed, further illuminating the need for a systematic approach to suture techniques.[3,16] Decreased nasal tip projection is a product of the suture being passed through the anterior medial crura and caudal septum at the nasal spine (**Fig. 13**). This also results in reducing the nasolabial angle and interdomal width.[14,16] These suture techniques may adjust the tip by increasing or decreasing projection by 3 mm to 4 mm, without the use of struts, grafts, or resection.[3]

Step 9: Rotation Control

The caudal margin placement of the interdomal suture rotates the lateral crura in the caudal direction and the opposite is true for a cephalic margin suture location. There is, however, a minimal shift produced in either direction.[16] The tip rotation suture is placed through the medial genu, or caudal to this point, and the caudal septum to effectively rotate the tip cephalad (**Fig. 14**). Widening and retraction of the lobule and columella also result if not previously secured with sutures.[16] Suture plication of the distal nasal septum to the proximal intercrural ligament with 5-0 PDS, allows tip rotation to a more cephalic position. This effectively reverses tip ptosis and has also been described in detail.[11]

Another tool is a rotation control graft of septal cartilage placed between the cephalad medial crus and the caudal septum. Similar to the columellar strut, both may increase or decrease the length of the membranous septal area and control the medial crural shape and position, while preventing columellar retraction with healing.[3] In the case of an over-rotated nasal tip, the DARTT graft is an extended dorsal spreader graft placed to stabilize the internal nasal valve patency while

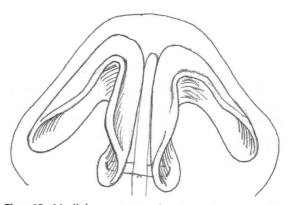

Fig. 13. Medial crura septal suture increases tip projection when placed though posterior medial crura footplates and caudal septum while decreasing projection when placed through anterior medial crura footplates and nasal spine.

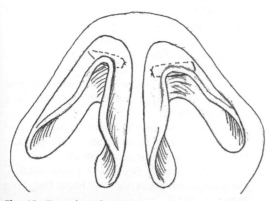

Fig. 12. Transdomal sutures.

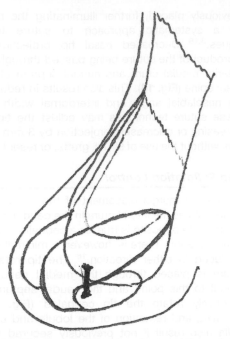

Fig. 14. The tip rotation suture is placed through the medial genu or caudal to this point and the caudal septum to effectively rotate the tip cephalad.

derotating the tip. The end result is a stronger dorsal septum and improved anterior septal angle.[1,11]

Step 10: Multiple Layered Closure

The SMAS surrounds the lower lateral crura and plays at least a minor role in tip support. Layered closure of the open rhinoplasty incision redistributes wound tension and decreases dead-space. SMAS reapproximation is essential to re-establishing and even increasing the integrity of the tip support.[11]

SUMMARY

Rhinoplasty remains a challenging art, but is now systematized at least in part, by recent understanding of the supporting mechanisms and how they may be manipulated to control the nasal tip. Nasal tip control is the key to a successful, aesthetically pleasing rhinoplasty result with preservation of nasal function.

ACKNOWLEDGMENTS

The authors wish to thank Cheryl Olomon, RN, for contributing all the drawings.

REFERENCES

1. Tardy EM, Thomas RJ. Ch 36: Rhinoplasty. In: Cummings otolaryngology head and neck surgery, 5th edition, vol. 1. Philadelphia. Mosby Elsevier; 2010. p. 509–44.
2. Behmand RA, Ghavami A, Guyuron B. Nasal tip sutures part I: the evolution. Plast Reconstr Surg 2003;112(4):1125–9 [discussion: 1146–9].
3. Tebbetts JB. Shaping and positioning the nasal tip without structural disruption: a new, systematic approach. Plast Reconstr Surg 1994;94(1):61–77.
4. Anderson JR. The dynamics of rhinoplasty, in Proceedings of the Ninth International Congress of Otolaryngology. Excerpta Medica International Congress Series, No. 206. Amsterdam: Excerpta Medica; 1969. p. 708–10.
5. Anderson JR. A reasoned approach to nasal base surgery. Arch Otolaryngol 1984;110(6):349–58.
6. Westreich RW, Lawson W. The tripod theory of nasal tip support revisited: the cantilevered spring model. Arch Facial Plast Surg 2008;10(3):170–9.
7. Johnson CM, Toriumi DM. Open structure rhinoplasty. Philadelphia: W.B. Saunders; 1990.
8. Janeke JB, Wright WK. Studies on the support of the nasal tip. Arch Otolaryngol 1971;93(5):458–64.
9. Tardy ME. Rhinoplasty: the art and science. Philadelphia: W.B. Saunders; 1997. p. 4.
10. Beaty MM, Dyer WK 2nd, Shawl MW. The quantification of surgical changes in nasal tip support. Arch Facial Plast Surg 2002;4(2):82–91.
11. Dyer WK 2nd. Nasal tip support and its surgical modification. Facial Plast Surg Clin North Am 2004; 12(1):1–13.
12. Nolst Trenite GJ. Surgery of the nasal tip: intranasal approach. In: Facial Plastic and Reconstructive Surgery, 3rd edition, New York: Thieme; 2009. p. 563–75.
13. Gruber RP, Nahai F, Bogdan MA, et al. Changing the convexity and concavity of nasal cartilages and cartilage grafts with horizontal mattress sutures: part I. Experimental results. Plast Reconstr Surg 2005;115(2):589–94.
14. Gruber RP, Nahai F, Bogdan MA, et al. Changing the convexity and concavity of nasal cartilages and cartilage grafts with horizontal mattress sutures: part II. Clinical results. Plast Reconstr Surg 2005;115(2): 595–606 [discussion: 607–8].
15. Dosanjh AS, Hsu C, Gruber RP. The hemitransdomal suture for narrowing the nasal tip. Ann Plast Surg 2010;64(6):708–12.
16. Guyuron B, Behmand RA. Nasal tip sutures part II: the interplays. Plast Reconstr Surg 2003; 112(4):1130–45 [discussion: 1146–9].
17. Corrado A, Bloom JD, Becker DG. Domal stabilization suture in tip rhinoplasty. Arch Facial Plast Surg 2009;11(3):194–7.

Dorsal Hump Surgery and Lateral Osteotomy

Behnam Bohluli, DMD[a],*, Nima Moharamnejad, DMD[b],
Mohammad Bayat, DMD[c]

KEYWORDS

- Dorsal hump • Surgery • Lateral osteotomy
- Cosmetic rhinoplasty

The presence of a prominent dorsal hump is one of the main reasons that patients seek cosmetic rhinoplasty. Dorsal surgery has been traditionally confined to simple hump trimming and leveling the nose in a profile view. Although modern concepts of dorsal surgery are based on the conservative reduction of excessive parts and the meticulous reconstruction and augmentation of deficient parts, special focus is usually made on internal valve function and making a pleasant esthetic brow line in the frontal view.

Lateral osteotomy is a controversial step in rhinoplasty, which is usually performed to narrow a wide nose, widen a narrow bony pyramid, straighten a deviated nose, or close an open roof deformity. The osteotomy is performed using several methods, although the internal continuous and external perforator are the main ways to perform the lateral osteotomy. Most other techniques are modifications of these basic methods.

The purpose of this article is to review the essential concepts of nasal hump surgery and lateral osteotomy as used in cosmetic rhinoplasty.

DORSAL NOSE SURGERY
Preoperative Analysis

A comprehensive preoperative analysis and proper diagnosis play the main roles in successful hump surgery; this evaluation usually starts with clinical examination of the nose. The bony pyramid is palpated to determine the length of nasal bones because it directly affects the treatment plan. For short nasal bones, hump resection is contraindicated or should be done conservatively, if ever. The thickness and consistency of the skin are sometimes important in determining the best graft material and method of dorsal augmentation. Internal nasal valve function should be examined carefully in case of valve incompetency because internal valve reinforcement might be considered even in the absence of a prominent nasal hump.

The importance of esthetic brow lines in dorsal surgery should be recognized. It is generally accepted that dorsal surgery has a great impact in making smooth, pleasing esthetic brow lines, which are formed by the 2 concave lines from the superior orbital rim and extending laterally toward the nasal tip (**Fig. 1**). The creation of these lines has a great impact on the final outcome of surgery in the frontal view. Obtaining a pleasant esthetic brow line is closely related to the internal valve reconstruction and should be considered for successful dorsal nasal surgery.

Classification of Dorsal Deformities and their Treatment Plan in an Algorithmic Approach

This classification is based on the need for hump removal and the amount of excessive hump determined during the preoperative analysis. The treatment plan will be based on the reduction of

[a] Department of Oral and Maxillofacial Surgery, Buali Hospital, Azad University, Neyestan #10, Pasdaran Avenue, Tehran, Iran
[b] Craniomaxillofacial Research Center, Shariati Hospital, Tehran University of Medical Sciences, Tehran, Iran
[c] Department of Oral and Maxillofacial Surgery, Shariati Hospital, Tehran University of Medical Sciences, Tehran, Iran
* Corresponding author.
E-mail address: bbohluli@yahoo.com

Oral Maxillofacial Surg Clin N Am 24 (2012) 75–86
doi:10.1016/j.coms.2011.10.005
1042-3699/12/$ – see front matter © 2012 Elsevier Inc. All rights reserved

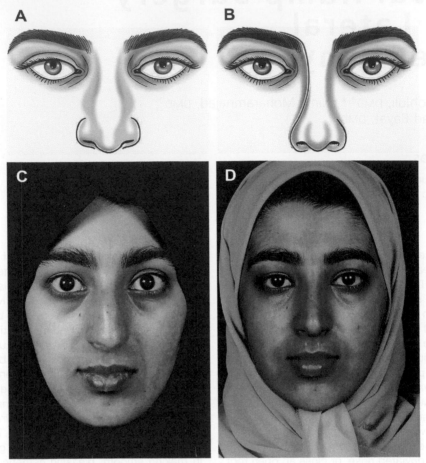

Fig. 1. (*A–D*) Esthetic brow lines are 2 imaginary concave lines that are drawn from superior orbital rim toward nasal tip [there is a lack of these lines in (*A*) and (*C*)].

excessive bony and cartilaginous segments and the augmentation areas of deficiency. Special emphasis is placed on the internal valve and the dorsal esthetic lines. In this classification, surgical techniques will start from simple composite resections to component resection with an autospreader flap; splay graft; and, finally, spreader grafts (**Fig. 2**). The authors generally prefer to use any excessive nasal tissue as flaps and to harvest septal or other donor sites for augmentation and reconstruction when an ideal result cannot be achieved via conservative (non–graft/flap) techniques. Dorsal surgery in more complicated rhinoplasty treatment plans may need special considerations that are discussed in a separate section.

Composite resection

This technique is simple and effective in patients with a straight (nondeviated) dorsum with minimal excessive hump (up to 2 mm of excess). This procedure may be done in both open and closed rhinoplasty approaches. In this technique, the

lower lateral cartilages are pushed downward by a double hook to have better access to the hump. The preplanned part of the cartilaginous septum is cut by a number 15 blade, then an osteotome is placed under the divided cartilaginous hump, the bony part is resected, and the excessive hump is taken out in 1 piece (**Figs. 3 and 4**). In this technique, care should be taken to preserve the mucosal lining underneath the junction of the upper lateral cartilages and nasal septum; the integrity of this mucosa prevents synechia formation and will work as spreaders to reinforce the valve and make pleasant esthetic brow lines postoperatively (**Figs. 5 and 6**).

The excised hump may be used as an effective autograft material that has been widely used for following indications:

1. Columella strut: The resected hump is cut and shaped as a strut. The bony part that is usually a small part of the graft is placed over the anterior nasal spine, and the cartilaginous segment

Bohluli-Moharamnejad dorsal nasal surgery algorithm

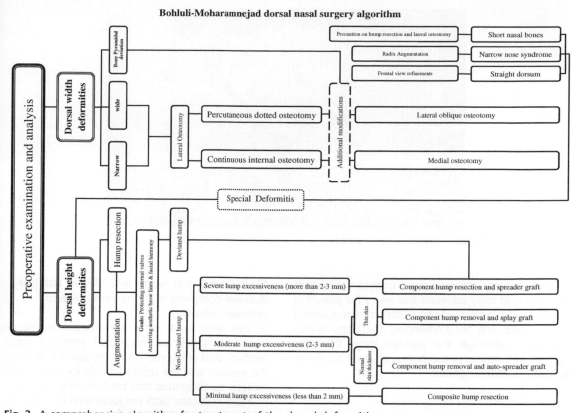

Fig. 2. A comprehensive algorithm for treatment of the dorsal deformities.

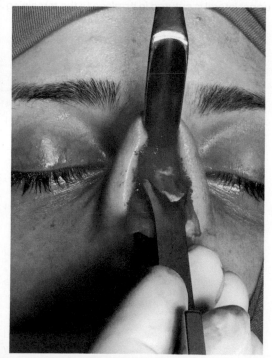

Fig. 3. Cartilaginous hump is cut by number 15 blades, then an osteotome is used to resect the bony part.

is inserted between 2 medial crura and fixed with sutures.

2. Tip graft: The cartilage may be separated from the bone and used as a tip graft.

3. To cover irregularity: As originally described by Skoog, in an overresected dorsum or inextremely thin skins with dorsal irregularities, the resected hump may be placed back to its original place to make a smooth dorsal surface.

4. Radix augmentation: In some patients, a combination of dorsal resection and radix augmentation is indicated. In these cases, composite resection is done, and then the resected part is trimmed and tailored as a graft material and placed back in a more cephalic position for radix augmentation (**Figs. 7–9**).

In case intraoperative judgments show that further hump removal is needed, upper lateral cartilages should be separated from the septum. After adjusting the dorsum, other measures of midvault reinforcements, such as spreader grafts, might be considered.

Technique modifications Some surgeons remove small bony humps by delicate rasps because they think rasping gives better control; however,

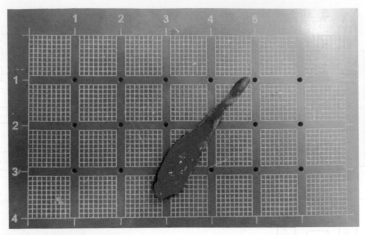

Fig. 4. Excessive hump is taken out in 1 piece.

a 1-piece hump removal gives considerable graft material and may alleviate the need for planning for a second graft donor site. Sometimes guarded osteotomes are recommended for bony hump resection, although the authors think that this type of osteotome is too bulky, at least for these delicate dorsal surgeries.

More than 2-mm hump resection in straight dorsum–component hump removal and autospreader flap

In this technique, after skeletonization, upper lateral cartilages are separated from the nasal septum, and lining mucosa is released both from the septum and the upper laterals for a few millimeters, cartilaginous and bony humps are incrementally resected until the ideal level is obtained, and then the edges of the upper lateral are grasped and folded inward to have the same level with the reduced septum (**Fig. 10**). The folded upper lateral is sutured in its place to the remaining

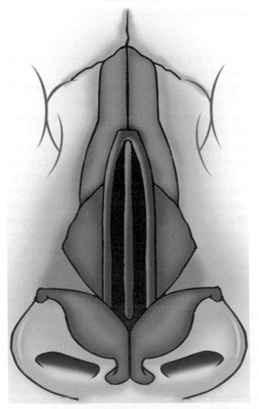

Fig. 5. Integrity of mucosa will prevent synechia and nasal valve collapse. Schematic view.

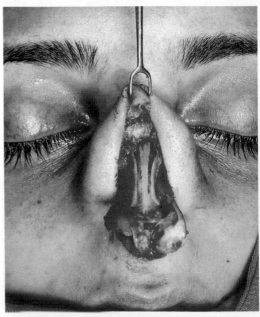

Fig. 6. Integrity of mucosa will prevent synechia and nasal valve collapse. Clinical view.

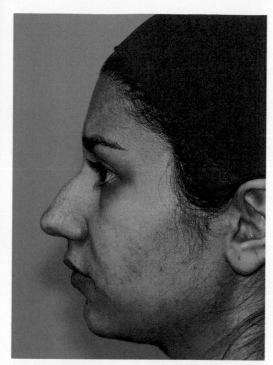

Fig. 7. In this patient, combination of resection and augmentation was indicated.

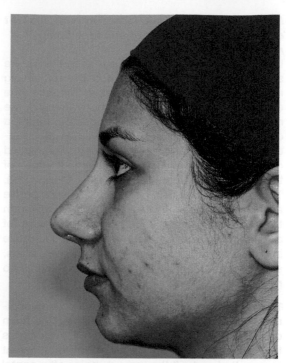

Fig. 9. In this patient, resected hump was replaced in dorsum in a more cephalic position.

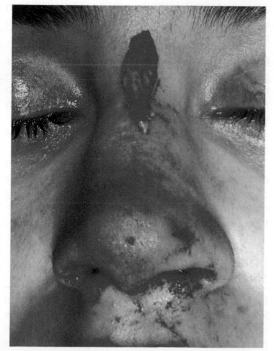

Fig. 8. In this patient, composite hump resection was performed.

intact upper lateral cartilage and fixed to the septum. Folded upper laterals may be hatched in the length of the autospreader flap to adjust the width of the dorsum and to get a better outline. The technique is completely reproducible and reversible, and if intraoperative judgments show an unpleasant appearance, sutures are easily removed, excessive parts of the upper lateral is conservatively trimmed, and the field would be ready for other classic augmentation techniques, such as spreader grafts.

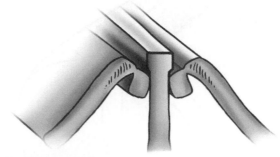

Fig. 10. Excessive upper lateral cartilages are folded in to preserve the support of nasal valve; a longitudinal incision is made over folded cartilage to adjust the width of dorsum.

More than 2-mm hump resection with straight dorsum and thin skins–component hump resection and splay grafts

In this technique, the upper lateral cartilages are separated from the septum and the underlying mucosa is dissected for a few millimeters, the cartilaginous hump and the bony humps are reduced, the upper lateral cartilages are trimmed conservatively, and then a rectangular piece of-crushed septal cartilage is refined and placed over the septal cartilage and between 2 edges of the upper lateral cartilages (**Figs. 11** and **12**). This method results in a smooth dorsal profile and may be efficient under thin skins, although this method needs a precise manipulation of a moldable graft material, which is not possible in all cases, and sometimes other treatment plans, such as spreader grafts, should be taken into mind.

Technical modifications Splay grafts were originally made from ear conchal cartilage; the main drawback of an ear cartilage graft for dorsum is the difficulty of manipulation and its inherent curves that make it the second choice after septal cartilage.

More than 2-mm hump resection deviated dorsum–component hump resection and spreader grafts

In this technique, 2 quadrangular pieces of septal cartilage are prepared, and these pieces are sutured to the septum on both sides (**Figs. 13–15**). The advent of the spreader graft is sometimes thought of as a revolution in straightening a dorsal deviation, which remains in the dorsal part of the septum after septoplasty. Although this technique is the gold standard of middle vault reconstruction after hump removal and may be used after all

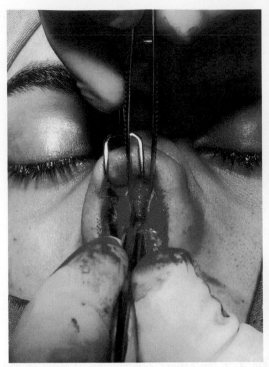

Fig. 12. Splay graft is a crushed piece of cartilage, which is placed over septum and under 2 upper lateral cartilages.

types of hump resection, the only drawback of spreader grafts is the need for a considerable amount of intact cartilage with good length, which is not always available, even in all primary esthetic nose surgeries.

Important points in using spreader grafts Spreader grafts may be used unilaterally or bilaterally, sometimes 2 or 3 pieces of grafts are used in one side to fill the deficient part of the dorsum or to straighten the deviated dorsal septum.

Spreader grafts may be extended under nasal bones to widen a narrow bony pyramid.

Spreader grafts are easily placed and fixed in an open-approach rhinoplasty, although these types of grafts are placed in a closed approach by making a tunnel between the upper lateral cartilage and the septum.

DORSAL SURGERY IN SPECIAL CASES
Short Nasal Bones

In normal bony pyramids, nasal bones cover at least half of the distance from the radix to the angle of the septum. In short nasal bones, the dorsal hump is almost entirely cartilaginous, and the resection of a cartilaginous roof endangers the midvault and significantly reduces the support of

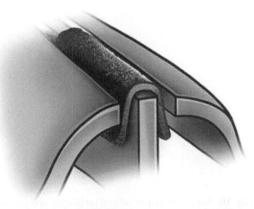

Fig. 11. Splay graft is a crushed piece of cartilage, which is placed over septum and under 2 upper lateral cartilages.

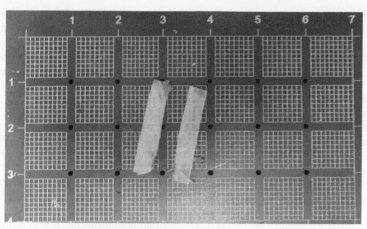

Fig. 13. Spreader graft is the quadrangular part of cartilage.

the upper lateral cartilages. If simultaneous lateral osteotomy is performed, the remaining support would be lost and the nose is in risk of severe collapse, which will have a disastrous result, both esthetically and functionally. Therefore, dorsal hump resection is contraindicated in short nasal bones. In cases of necessity, it should be done conservatively, and midvault reinforcement should be strongly considered.

Narrow Nose Syndrome

These patients usually have a prominent hump and an overprojected narrow midvault and low radix. Palpation of the bony pyramid shows extremely small nasal bones. Dorsal surgery in these patients is usually a combination of cartilaginous hump trimming, spreader grafts, and precise radix augmentation. Crushed septal cartilage is the material of choice in radix augmentation, although trimmed or crushed conchal cartilage may be used

with caution. Temporalis fascia is also effective in limited radix augmentations; temporalis fascia is sometimes used to cover the cartilage grafts in thin skins.

Straight Dorsum

In these patients, the dorsum is straight or with small irregularity. Dorsal surgery is usually limited to minimal or no hump resection. The main efforts could be made to create a pleasant frontal view.

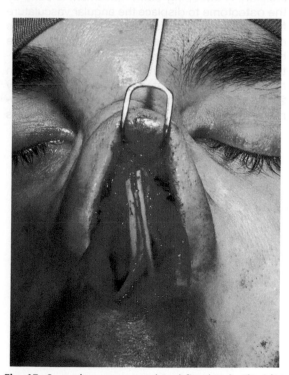

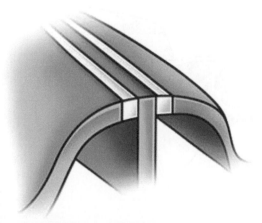

Fig. 14. Spreaders are sutured and fixed to both sides of dorsum.

Fig. 15. Spreaders are sutured and fixed to both sides of dorsum.

Insisting on reductive surgery may result in disastrous outcomes.

LATERAL OSTEOTOMY

Lateral osteotomy is a controversial step in rhinoplasty that is usually performed to narrow a wide nose to widen a narrow bony pyramid, to straighten a deviated nose, and to close an open roof deformity. This procedure may be performed in 3 levels (low to low, low to high, and high to high), which shows the pathway of the osteotomy line from the pyriform aperture toward the medial canthus. Many methods and instruments are introduced to obtain better and more predictable results. Unilateral-guarded osteotomies; bilateral-guarded osteotomies; nasal saws; rhinotom; and motor-driven instruments, such as piezosurgery devices, are among the most common used tools, although there are 2 main ways in performing an osteotomy, internal continuous and external perforator, which are discussed in detail.

Percutaneous Dotted Osteotomy

In this technique, a straight 2-mm osteotome is used to perform the osteotomy. First a stab incision is made in the nasofacial skin. This incision is usually located in the midway of the osteotomy line. Then the osteotome is inserted through the incision. A sweeping-down movement is done by the osteotome to displace the angular vasculature from the osteotomy site. It is thought that this maneuver may reduce the risk of intraoperative bleeding and postoperative ecchymosis. The osteotomy is started from the pyriform aperture, an osteotomy hole is created, and it is repeated every 2 to 3 mm toward the medial canthus in a perforating manner (**Fig. 16**). Then the nasal bone is

medialized by light finger pressure. Failing to medialize the nasal bone shows either the osteotomy is not complete or a lateral oblique osteotomy should be added to the first osteotomy line and more heavy pressure should not be exerted.

Lateral Oblique Osteotomy

Lateral oblique osteotomy is an external alternative of classical medial osteotomy. It is usually performed to help medialize extremely wide bony nasal walls, to prevent any uncontrolled bony fracture during mobilization of the nasal bones, and to prevent rocker deformity. For performing a lateral oblique osteotomy, a skin marker is used to draw a line from the cephalic ending point of the lateral osteotomy line toward the dorsum. This line has an angle of 15° to 30° to the lateral osteotomy line. Then, a small stab incision is made over the medial canthus on the midway of the drawn line. A 2-mm chisel is inserted, and the osteotomy is performed in a dotted manner (**Fig. 17**). This technique is generally performed in completing an external perforating osteotomy, although the lateral oblique osteotomy is extensively used in conjunction with an intranasal continuous osteotomy instead of an intranasal medial osteotomy.

Important points in percutaneous perforating osteotomy

1. Infracture is done by light finger pressure and heavy pressure or extreme right and left movements of bony fragments should be avoided.
2. A 2-mm chisel should have an angle with the bone during the osteotomy (**Fig. 18**). Using a full cutting edge of osteotome may scatter the bone or make an undesired fracture line.

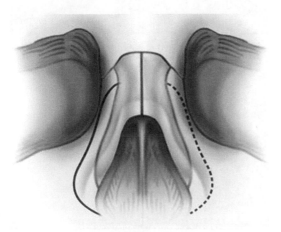

Fig. 16. External perforator osteotomy in left and internal continuous in right side.

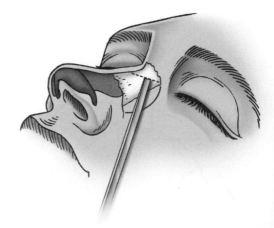

Fig. 17. Lateral oblique osteotomy starts from medial canthus and ends in dorsum in a doted manner.

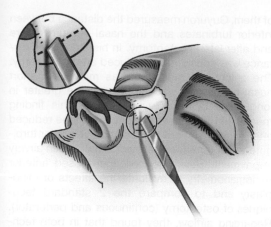

Fig. 18. Cutting edge of 2-mm osteotome is not in complete contact with bone. By this angulation, osteotomy holes are easily made, and the risk of bone scattering is reduced.

3. After infracture of both the left and right sides, a light finger pressure is held for a short time to control bleeding. A cold, normal saline rinse would be beneficial during this period of time.

Technical modifications

Perforating osteotomy is sometimes performed through a small intranasal incision instead of skin incisions.

Continuous Internal Osteotomy

In intranasal osteotomy, a small mucosal incision is made in the pyriform aperture, then a guarded 2- to 4-mm osteotome is introduced through the incision, and with tap strokes of a mallet, the osteotomy is started from the pyriform aperture toward the medial canthus (see **Fig. 16**). The cephalic extent of the osteotomy line should not be extended from medial canthus.

Medial Osteotomy

Medial osteotomy has traditionally been performed for further mobilization of nasal bones and makes a narrower nose. In current concepts of rhinoplasty, there is no tendency to make an excessively narrow and small nose, so this technique should be preserved for its few indications that are mentioned as follows:

1. Deviated bony pyramid
2. Excessively wide bony base
3. To widen a nose and make space for putting spreader grafts
4. When the dorsum is not resected or the amount was not enough to open the dorsal roof.

Surgical technique: a straight osteotome is inserted between the upper lateral cartilage, and then the osteotome is angled 15° to the sagittal plane (**Fig. 19**). The osteotomy is started with tap strokes of a mallet. It is continued cephalically up to the medial canthus. If excessive narrowing is desired, a small wedge of nasal bone that is in contact to septum must be resected. A 15° angulation of the osteotomy obeys normal cleavage lines in nasal bone fractures and will prevent the insertion of the osteotome to the thick bones of the radix. This maneuver is usually performed to complete the internal continuous osteotomy, but it may also be used in conjunction with an external perforated osteotomy.

Important points in continuous osteotomy

1. Subperiosteal dissection and making a tunnel for guarded osteotome makes a dead space that may be filled with hematoma and granulation tissue, additionally it reduces the stability of bony fragments and should be avoided
2. Infracture should be performed with light pressure excessive movements should be avoided
3. By using a curved osteotome, a small triangle of bone in the pyriform area will remain (**Fig. 20**). Webster thinks this bony triangle will preserve the internal nasal valve from excessive narrowing and will preserve airway patency as much as possible.

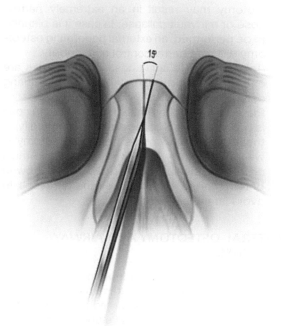

Fig. 19. Medial osteotomy is usually performed with 15° angulations to avoid thick bone in radix area.

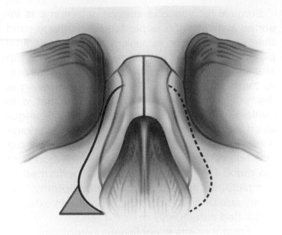

Fig. 20. A small wedge of bone is usually preserved in pyriform aperture. This triangle will prevent excessive narrowing of dorsum in internal valve area.

4. Mobilizing fractured bones by lifting or turning the handle of the osteotome after the osteotomy is extremely traumatic and may result in the luxation of bones or the collapse of bony vault and, logically, should be avoided.

Contraindications of lateral osteotomy: Lateral osteotomy is not beneficial in all rhinoplasty patients. The following are the main known groups that lateral osteotomy should be avoided in or performed with extreme caution:

1. Short nasal bones: In these patients, lateral osteotomy may result in an extremely narrow nose or midvault collapse. In case it is planned to be performed, an external perforating osteotomy will give better control and stability.
2. Aging noses: In aging noses, nasal bones are extremely fragile and may be scattered during osteotomy.
3. Platyrrhine: In these patients, the tip of the nose is bulky and nasal bones are short. Generally, in these type of the noses, lateral osteotomy is well tolerated by bony pyramid and the main problem is the harmony of bulky tip to narrowed bony pyramid, which makes the surgeons to avoid lateral osteotomy.

LATERAL OSTEOTOMY AND AIRWAY CHANGES

The main result of lateral osteotomy in most cases would be medialization of lateral nasal walls. This movement may potentially reduce the airway capacity of the nose. Several studies with controversial results have assessed the effects of rhinoplasty on the airway, but lateral osteotomy was the main concern of the study in only a few

of them. Guyuron measured the distance between inferior turbinates and the nasal septum before and after lateral osteotomy. In his study, this distance was considerably reduced after osteotomy. The amount of reduction was minimal in short nasal bones and was reported to be greater in long nasal bones. Guyuron thinks this finding means that total airway capacity may be reduced after rhinoplasty, but the distance of inferior turbinate to septum does not necessarily mean airway impairment. Helal and colleagues used anterior rhinomanometry to evaluate the effects of rhinoplasty and to compare the 2 standard techniques of osteotomy (continuous and perforator). Regarding airflow, they found that in both techniques airflow is significantly reduced. In comparing 2 techniques, there was no significant difference between an external perforating osteotomy and an internal continuous osteotomy. In contrast, Coutriss and Goldwyn used anterior rhinomanometry in their large series of rhinoplasty patients, and their findings did not show any adverse effect on the airway after rhinoplasty. They think these controversial results are in some extent caused by the inherent limitations of rhinomanometry and are related to techniques of rhinoplasty. In Byrne study, external perforating osteotomy and internal continuous osteotomies were performed in fresh cadavers with short nasal bones. The results were compared by anatomic dissections. This study showed that internal continuous osteotomy disrupted the periosteum on both sides of the osteotomy and made a considerable narrowing of the nasal valves that is not usually desired in these types of noses. All these studies, and other similar studies, with all their controversial results show that nasal airway changes in rhinoplasty are extremely complex and may not be clarified by available data. Although it is generally accepted that lateral osteotomy may potentially endanger the nasal airway, some surgeons think they can compensate these possible adverse effects by precise management of septal deviations and reinforcement of external and internal nasal valves, some others suggest turbinate surgery to enhance the nasal airway, although it seems that meticulous techniques of lateral osteotomy, trying to make a predictable bone fracture and finally avoiding osteotomy in contraindicated cases would minimize the risk of airway damages.

CHOOSING THE OSTEOTOMY TECHNIQUE IN RHINOPLASTY

Many studies have compared 2 standard methods of osteotomy. It is mostly thought that, in internal continuous osteotomy, the possibility of mucosal tearing and periosteal disruption would be higher, which may cause intraoperative bleeding and postoperative edema, although the importance of this finding in the final result of an osteotomy is not clear. It is also thought that postoperative ecchymosis is larger in internal osteotomy. On the other hand, a visible scar is a potential risk in the external perforating technique, although many studies have ruled out this possibility.

Incomplete fracture and mobilization and the need for repeating the osteotomy procedure several times is another potential drawback of external perforator osteotomy. Finally, it seems that the final results of osteotomy extremely depend on the skills and experience of the surgeon because none of the aforementioned studies have convinced the rhinoplasty surgeons to unanimously leave one technique and accept the other.

Changing the Osteotomy Technique During the Operation

Both the continuous and perforator techniques have their potentials and limitations. A rhinoplasty surgeon usually chooses one of the standard osteotomy techniques and gets experience and skills on it, but it is generally suggested to be familiar with both methods to change the osteotomy technique in special conditions and use the advantages of both techniques.

Switching from external perforator to internal continuous: In the perforator technique, small osteotomy dots are made in the osteotomy line. Then these dots are connected by light finger pressure. In some cases with thick bones or aging noses, infracture does not happen on the first try. Repeating the osteotomy with the same technique may be traumatic and ineffective. It is generally suggested to change the osteotomy technique and use the internal continuous method.

Switching from internal continuous to external perforator: Internal continuous osteotomy is a blind technique and sometimes osteotomy lines do not exactly pass the desired plans or an unpredicted fracture line happens. In these cases, repeating the internal continuous technique may worsen the situation, and the use of a 2-mm osteotome with the external perforator method may easily restore the fracture line.

SUMMARY

Dorsal hump surgery and lateral osteotomy are important steps in rhinoplasty. Currently, dorsal surgery has found a great relation with the reconstruction of internal valve and creating esthetic brow lines.

Lateral osteotomy remains a challenge in rhinoplasty, although some basic principals are generally accepted: Firstly, the indications are to narrow a wide nose; to widen a narrow nose; to close an open roof; and, finally, to straighten a deviated bone. Second, it may be performed in 3 levels (low to low, low to high, and high to low), which show a pathway of the osteotome from the pyriform aperture to the medial canthus. Finally, there are 2 main ways for performing the osteotomy that are both effective. A surgeon may find one method as the method of choice but should be familiar with the other to use advantages of both techniques.

FURTHER READINGS

Bohluli B. External versus internal osteotomy in rhinoplasty. In: abstracts of the 18th International Conference on Oral and Maxillofacial Surgery. Int J Oral Maxillofac Surg 2007;36(11):972–3.

Bohluli B, Sarkarat F, Ashtiani AK, et al. Selecting the osteotome in rhinoplasty. Aesthet Surg J 2009;29(4):335.

Byrd HS, Meade RA, Gonyon DL Jr. Using the autospreader flap in primary rhinoplasty. Plast Reconstr Surg 2007;119(6):1897–902.

Byrne PJ, Walsh WE, Hilger PA. The use of "inside-out" lateral osteotomies to improve outcome in rhinoplasty. Arch Facial Plast Surg 2003;5(3):251–5.

Coutriss EH, Goldwyn RM. The effects of nasal surgery on airflow. Plast Reconstr Surg 1983;72(1):9–21.

Erişir F, Tahamiler R. Lateral osteotomies in rhinoplasty: a safer and less traumatic method. Aesthet Surg J 2008;28(5):518–20.

Ford CN, Battaglia DG, Gentry LR. Preservation of periosteal attachment in lateral osteotomy. Ann Plast Surg 1984;13(2):107–11.

Gruber R, Chang TN, Kahn D, et al. Broad nasal bone reduction: an algorithm for osteotomies. Plast Reconstr Surg 2007;119(3):1044–53.

Gruber RP, Perkins SW. Humpectomy and spreader flaps. Clin Plast Surg 2010;37(2):285–91.

Gruber RP, Park E, Newman J, et al. The spreader flap in primary rhinoplasty. Plast Reconstr Surg 2007;119(6):1903–10.

Gryskiewicz JM, Gryskiewicz KM. Nasal osteotomies: a clinical comparison of the perforating methods versus the continuous technique. Plast Reconstr Surg 2004;113(5):1445–56 [discussion: 1457–8].

Gryskiewicz JM. Visible scars from percutaneous osteotomies. Plast Reconstr Surg 2005;116(6):1771–5.

Guyuron B, Michelow BJ, Englebardt C. Upper lateral splay graft. Plast Reconstr Surg 1998;102(6):2169–77.

Guyuron B. Nasal osteotomy and airway changes. Plast Reconstr Surg 1998;102(3):856–60 [discussion: 861–3].

Harshbarger RJ, Sullivan PK. Lateral nasal osteotomies: implications of bony thickness on fracture patterns. Ann Plast Surg 1999;42(4):365–70 [discussion: 370–1].

Helal MZ, El-Tarabishi M, Magdy Sabry S, et al. Effects of rhinoplasty on the internal nasal valve: a comparison between internal continuous and external perforating osteotomy. Ann Plast Surg 2010;64(5): 649–57.

Hinton AE, Hung T, Daya H, et al. Visibility of puncture sites after external osteotomy in rhinoplastic surgery. Arch Facial Plast Surg 2003;5(5):408–11.

Kuran I, Ozcan H, Usta A, et al. Comparison of four different types of osteotomes for lateral osteotomy: a cadaver study. Aesthetic Plast Surg 1996;20(4): 323–6.

Lejour M, Duchateau J, Potaznik A. Routine reinsertion of the hump in rhinoplasty. Scand J Plast Reconstr Surg 1986;20(1):55–9.

Regnault P, Alfaro A. The Skoog rhinoplasty: a modified technique. Plast Reconstr Surg 1980;66(4):578–90.

Rohrich RJ, Hollier LH. Use of spreader grafts in the external approach to rhinoplasty. Clin Plast Surg 1996;23(2):255–62.

Rohrich RJ, Janis JE, Adams WP, et al. An update on the lateral nasal osteotomy in rhinoplasty: an anatomic endoscopic comparison of the external versus the internal approach. Plast Reconstr Surg 2003; 111(7):2461–2 [discussion: 2463].

Rohrich RJ, Krueger JK, Adams WP Jr, et al. Achieving consistency in the lateral nasal osteotomy during rhinoplasty: an external perforated technique. Plast Reconstr Surg 2001;108(7):2122–30 [discussion: 2131–2].

Rohrich RJ, Minoli JJ, Adams WP, et al. The lateral nasal osteotomy in rhinoplasty: an anatomic endoscopic comparison of the external versus the internal approach. Plast Reconstr Surg 1997;99(5):1309–12 [discussion: 1313].

Rohrich RJ, Muzaffar AR, Janis JE. Component dorsal hump reduction: the importance of maintaining dorsal aesthetic lines in rhinoplasty. Plast Reconstr Surg 2004;114(5):1298–308 [discussion: 1309–12].

Sheen JH. Rhinoplasty: personal evolution and milestones. Plast Reconstr Surg 2000;105(5):1820–52 [discussion: 1853].

Sheen JH. Spreader graft: a method of reconstructing the roof of the middle nasal vault following rhinoplasty. Plast Reconstr Surg 1984;73(2):230–9.

Skoog T. A method of hump reduction in rhinoplasty. A technique for preservation of the nasal roof. Arch Otolaryngol 1966;83(3):283–7.

Webster RC, Davidson TM, Smith RC. Curved lateral osteotomy for airway protection in rhinoplasty. Arch Otolaryngol 1977;103(8):454–8.

Nasal Base Surgery

Behnam Bohluli, DMD[a],*, Nima Moharamnejad, DMD[b],
Amin Yamani, DMD[c]

KEYWORDS

- Nasal base • Ethnic variation • Rhinoplasty
- Orthognathic surgery

The nasal base is an important aspect of the nose with a complex anatomic architecture comprising a combination of cartilages, skin, connective tissues, and ligaments; it forms the external nasal valve and plays an important role in nasal airway function. The history of nasal base surgery dates back to 1892 when Weird introduced his technique of resection of a small wedge of the alar skin. For nearly 100 years all the techniques and modifications were aimed at finding a way for resection of a wider volume of skin and concealing scar lines in normal grooves and creases. However, some recent studies show that all the nasal base deformities cannot be corrected by simple excision and suturing techniques. Alar release and medialization would be effective in some of these deformities.

This article presents an overview of conventional concepts of alar base surgeries, which have remained unchanged over many years. Indications and limitations of each technique are discussed, followed by a more detailed description of alar release and medialization.

ANATOMIC EVALUATION OF NASAL BASE

The nasal base forms an equilateral triangle that consists of two pear-shaped nostrils. These two nostrils have their long axis 45° to the long axis of the columella, and form two-thirds of the length of the nasal base. The columella is located between the two nostrils and ideally should form two-thirds of the height of the nasal base, and should be nearly equal to the length of the upper lip. The form of the columella is directly affected by divergences or flaring of two medial crura and the amount of connective tissue between them. The area above the nostrils is called the tip lobule, which comprises one-third to one-half of the height of the nasal base; the alar crease or alar facial groove is the junction between the nose and face, The amount of alar tissue that extends from the alar crease is called alar flare. The width of the nasal base is usually the distance between two alar flares, and this width should ideally fall within 2 mm of the lines that are drawn vertically from the medial canthus. The nasal sill is an area located between the nasofacial groove and the columella (**Fig. 1**).

Regarding the plane of the alar lobule, the axis of the alar lobule, as defined by Sheen, is the position of the vertical plane of the alar lobule relative to the horizontal plane of the nasal base in frontal view; this plane is optimally slightly divergent. Excessive divergence shows that excessive flare exists and that alar medialization should be planed; in some patients this plane is oriented vertically, which shows that alar base resection is contraindicated and may result in a disproportionally narrow base (**Fig. 2**).

Ethnic Variations in Nasal Base Anatomy

Nasal base anatomy in different genders is extensively discussed in the literature; Farkas defined 5 different nostril types in different ethnic nasal bases that were based on nostril orientation (**Fig. 3**). Standard values are usually defined based on anthropometric measurements in the normal Caucasian female face. In African Americans the projection of the tip is generally lower. The

[a] Department of Oral and Maxillofacial Surgery, Buali Hospital, Azad University, Neyestan #10, Pasdaran Avenue, Tehran, Iran
[b] Craniomaxillofacial Research Center, Shariati Hospital, Tehran University of Medical Sciences, Tehran, Iran
[c] Department of Oral and Maxillofacial Surgery, Buali Hospital, Azad University, Tehran, Iran
* Corresponding author.
E-mail address: bbohluli@yahoo.com

Oral Maxillofacial Surg Clin N Am 24 (2012) 87–94
doi:10.1016/j.coms.2011.10.009
1042-3699/12/$ – see front matter © 2012 Elsevier Inc. All rights reserved.

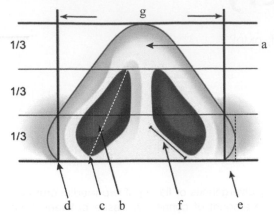

Fig. 1. Nasal tip lobule is the area above the nostrils, which makes up one-third to one-half of the height of the nasal base (a); nostrils (b) have an angulation of 45° to the long axis of the columella (c); the junction of nasal skin and cheek is the nasofacial groove (d); the amount of tissue that extends from the nasofacial groove is alar flare (e); the area between the nasofacial groove and columella is the nasal sill (f); and the distance between two alar flares is the nasal width (g).

columella is short and nostrils round. The interalar to intercanthal ratio is 1.25:1 in females and 1.3:1 in males; the nasal base is therefore relatively short and excessive alar flaring exists.

In Middle Eastern noses support of lower lateral cartilages is weak. Mild alar flaring, nostril asymmetry, large ala, and widened alar base are commonly encountered. Conservative alar base surgery is usually indicated in this group of patients.

In Asian noses the interalar distance is generally wider than the intercanthal distance. Severe alar flare and horizontally oriented nostrils are commonly seen.

PREOPERATIVE EVALUATION

Preoperative evaluation usually starts with a comprehensive interview with rhinoplasty candidates. Any history of massive scar or keloid formation may affect the treatment plan. The importance of the external nasal valve should be emphasized, and overzealous excision of nostrils must be avoided. The external nasal valve must be closely observed during deep breathing; partial or complete valve incompetency demands special concern in nasal base surgeries. All the ethnical and cultural characteristics should be borne in mind, as dogmatic plans for reductive alar base excisions may result in dissatisfaction. Tissue excisions in nasal base surgery, in contrast to other rhinoplasty maneuvers, are irreversible. Life-size photography is an integral part of preoperative evaluations. Photographic analysis should be done in at least in two directions, frontal and basal views being the minimum requirement for a thorough photographic evaluation. Deep-breathing photography easily documents most of the external nasal valve incompetence and may be added to the routine preoperative photo series.

DYNAMIC CHANGES IN NASAL BASE ANATOMY DURING RHINOPLASTY

The width of the nasal base may change considerably in some tip-plasty maneuvers, as during de-projecting techniques alar width and alar flare may increase; conversely, in a projecting nasal tip the width of nasal base is decreased, and structural grafting techniques such as alar contouring grafts and lateral crural strut grafts may potentially increase alar flare (**Fig. 4**). Some of these potential changes may be predicted preoperatively and be

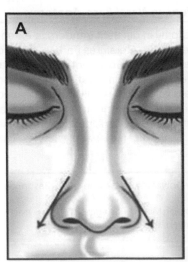
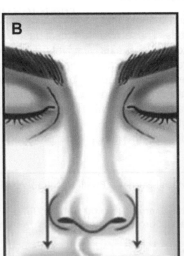
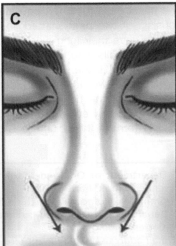

Fig. 2. Axis of alar lobule may be vertical (*A*), divergent (*B*), and convergent (*C*).

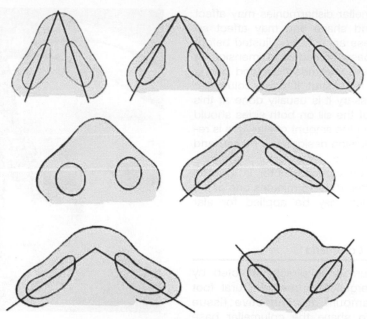

Fig. 3. Ethnic variations in nostril axis. (*Data from* Farkas LG, Hreczko TA, Deutsch CK. Objective assessment of standard nostril types—a morphometric study. Ann Plast Surg 1983;11(5):381–9.)

considered in the treatment plan for nasal base surgery, though frequent intraoperative judgments are necessary to obtain the best results; if any doubt exists the nasal base surgery may be postponed or a second office-based surgery under local anesthesia carried out a few weeks or months after initial surgery.

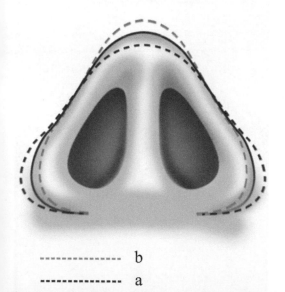

-------------- b

-------------- a

Fig. 4. Nasal width and flare may change during rhinoplasty. If the nose is deprojected, width and flare increase (a) and when projection increases, width and flare decrease (b).

NASAL BASE CONSIDERATIONS IN SIMULTANEOUS RHINOPLASTY AND ORTHOGNATHIC SURGERY

Simultaneous orthognathic surgery and rhinoplasty is frequently performed by oral and maxillofacial surgeons. It is generally accepted that LeFort I osteotomy widens the nasal base and increases alar flares. Widening of the alar base may occur in all types of LeFort I osteotomies, but is more often seen in LeFort I impactions and anterior advancements. These changes are beneficial in some patients with narrow noses, but may attenuate the situation in cases with poor tip support and wide nasal bases. Many procedures are performed to overcome these effects; first an effort is made to form a new wider bed by trimming the anterior nasal spine and/or pyriform aperture and lowering the floor of the nose to make enough space for facial soft tissues in their new skeletal framework. The effects and stability of alar cinch suture in reorientation of widened alar walls after LeFort osteotomies is extremely controversial; however, in cases of necessity it may be done through alar base incisions.

OPERATIVE TECHNIQUES IN NASAL BASE SURGERY

Alar base surgery is usually the final step in rhinoplasty. A caliper is used to recheck all the dimensions. Columellar disharmonies may affect the nostril size and shape and may affect sill dimensions, so these are usually adjusted before any other nasal base procedure. Dimension of columellar width is sometimes corrected during fixation of the columellar strut. If further columellar correction is necessary it is usually done at this stage. The width of the sill on both sides should be determined, then the amount of alar flare is re-assessed. Next, incision designs are planed and incision lines are marked by surgical pens, then local anesthetic with vasoconstrictor is injected in incision lines. After 10 to 15 minutes one of the following techniques may be applied for alar base surgery.

Narrowing Wide Columella

The width of columella is directly affected by distance and divergence of medial crural foot plates and the amount of connective tissue between them. To shape the columellar base a stab incision is made on both lateral sides of columellar base. A horizontal mattress suture is performed through two stab incisions; the suture is tightened gradually and tied when a suitable width of columella is achieved, then the stab incisions are closed with 6-0 nylon suture. This maneuver will affect the surface and orientation of nostrils (**Figs. 5–7**).

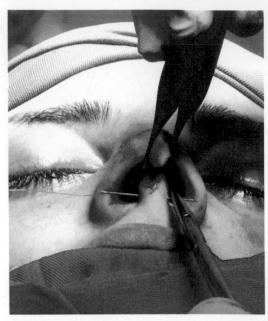

Fig. 6. Two stab incisions are made on both sides of the columella, and a mattress suture is done using a straight needle.

Wedge Resection

In this technique a small wedge of skin is resected from lateral aspect of alar skin. The inferior border of incision must be located in the nasofacial

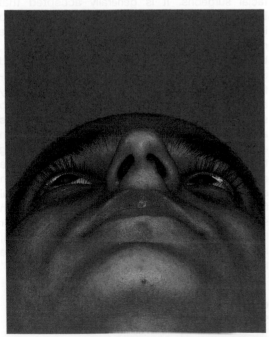

Fig. 5. Columellar deformities may affect nostril shape and orientation.

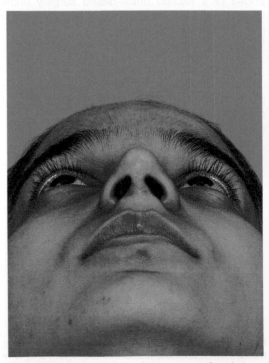

Fig. 7. Postoperative view of the same patient in basal view.

groove, and the superior border may be placed up to 3 mm over inferior to the incision line. Incisions are usually started with a no. 11 blade then continued with a no. 15 blade. Care should be taken not to enter vestibular linings. Incision lines are sutured with 6-0 nylon sutures. In wedge resection all efforts are made to hide the incisions in normal creases and shadows of the nose. Care must be taken during the procedure to ensure a minimal amount of skin should be excised, bearing in mind the possibility of visible scarring (**Fig. 8**).

Indications for wedge resection

1. *To reduce excessive alar flare.* Alar flare is the amount of alar tissue that extends from the na- sofacial groove; excessive alar tissue is some- times diagnosed in preoperative analysis or occurs in deprojecting procedures.
2. *To refine thick bulky alar tissue.* In bulky nasal walls the nostrils are usually small, so refining procedures are usually planned to reduce the tissues without entering the nasal sill and vesti- bule. In this technique the lateral nasal wall is refined without the size and shape of nostrils being affected.
3. *To reduce the height of the lateral nasal wall.* This technique reduces the height of lateral nasal walls, but should not be replaced by known standard deprojecting methods.

Important points in wedge resection

Incision lines are usually hidden in the nasofacial groove, although in a modification that was defined by Sheen, the inferior incision line is placed 1 mm superior to the nasofacial groove to conceal the scar in normal nasal shadows and make a curved, agreeable alar wall.

A normal flaring nostril is much more pleasing in appearance than a visible scar and distorted nasal base, therefore the amount of excised tissue should be minimal and closure should be done meticulously without any tension.

Nostril Sill Resection

If the nasal base is too wide or the circumference of nostrils is large, sill resection is indicated. In this technique two parallel markings are made in the nostril sill, then this small part of sill is resected. The incision lines are precisely sutured with 6-0 nylon sutures (**Fig. 9**).

Important points in nostril sill resection
In most cases incision lines do not enter the nasal vestibule; vestibular incisions are rarely indicated when there is a plan to reduce the size of nostrils.

Sill resection does not diminish excessive flare, and this problem should be solved by wedge resection or alar medialization.

Incisions should not enter medially to the colu- mellar base, otherwise notching or distortion may occur. Asymmetric alar bases may be corrected by unequal excision of alar base tissue on two sides.

Combination of Wedge and Sill Resection

In some patients both excessive flare and wide nasal base are seen. In these cases a combination of wedge and sill excision may be used (**Fig. 10**).

Lateral Wall Debulking (Rim Excision)

When lateral nasal walls of the nose are thick and bulky, debulking procedures are indicated. To perform this technique an elliptical surface of

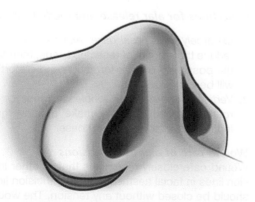

Fig. 8. Wedge resection. Two parallel incisions are made in the lateral nasal wall. Incision line may be placed in nasofacial groove or up to 1 mm above it.

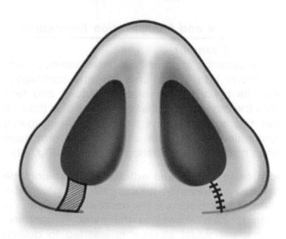

Fig. 9. For sill resection, two parallel incisions are made in the nostril sill; a small part of the sill is re- sected and meticulously sutured.

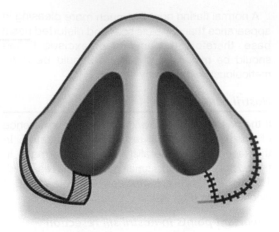

Fig. 10. When both excessive alar flare and sill exist, wedge and sill excisions are combined.

medial alar wall is marked and excised with a wedge-type incision. Incision lines usually are based on normal rim incisions and are easily closed with 6-0 nylon sutures.

Cinch Suture (Alar Release and Medialization)

In 1981 Millard first described this method for correcting wide flat nostrils in normal rhinoplasty patients. He used a circumferential nonresorbable suture through alar base incisions to medialize flared alar walls. The main drawback of this technique was recurrence and scar formation. Re-advent of this technique goes back to 2008, when Rohrich performed a comprehensive anatomic study on the pyriform area and explained the role of pyriform ligament in translating shape and position of alar walls. This study was the basis for more laboratory and clinical research.

Alar Release and Medialization Techniques

Pyriform ligament
This ligament originates from nasal bones, covers the lower lateral and upper lateral cartilages, extends toward the pyriform aperture, and reaches the other side at the nasal spine. It is thought that this ligament plays the main role in spatial positioning of alar walls, and should be released when massive medialization is required (**Fig. 11**).

Surgical technique and indications This technique is usually performed through sill incisions. After performing incisions in the nasal sill, dissection is done to gain access to the pyriform aperture, then a periosteal elevator is inserted to detach the pyriform ligament both inside and outside of the pyriform aperture and anterior maxilla. Each alar wall is medialized by a circumferential suture

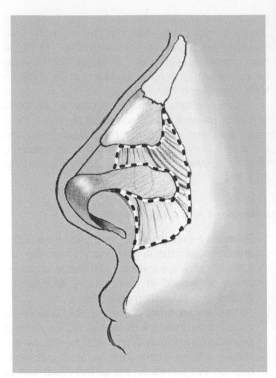

Fig. 11. The boundaries of the pyriform ligament show the superior border at the nasal bone and the inferior border at the anterior nasal spine. Dotted line displays the limits of this fascial network. (*Data from* Rohrich RJ, Hoxworth RE, Thornton JF, et al. The pyriform ligament. Plast Reconstr Surg 2008;121(1): 277–81.)

that starts from the dermis of the alar incision, goes though the nasal base and columella, and enters the other sill incision site before turning back to the original site. The same steps are done for the other alar wall, then sutures are gradually tightened and the alar walls medialized by these sutures (**Fig. 12**).

Indications for alar release and medialization

1. *Extremely wide nasal base.* Alar release could reduce the amount of resected tissue, therefore the possibility of scar formation and distortion will be decreased.
2. *Vertically oriented alar lobule.* In these cases routine procedures may make a convergent lobule and distort the nasal base.

Wound care of alar base incisions
Wound care closely resembles that of other incision lines in facial aesthetic surgery. Incision lines should be closed without any tension. The wound may be continuously rinsed during suturing time; this maneuver removes any possible fibrin clots and may help scar-free healing. The wounds are

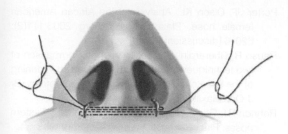

Fig. 12. In alar release and medialization, classic sill incisions are made with resection of a small part of tissue, or without resection two circumferential sutures are done to medialize alar walls after releasing pyriform ligament and perialar soft tissue. The first suture picks up dermis tissue of alar wall and passes through the nasal base and columella until it appears in the second sill incision area, then it returns back to its original site. Exactly the same procedure is done for the second side. Two sutures are gradually tightened to medialize the two side walls in a symmetric position. (*Data from* Gruber RP, Freeman MB, Hsu C, et al. Nasal base reduction by alar release: a laboratory evaluation. Plast Reconstr Surg 2009;123(2):709–15; and Gruber RP, Freeman MB, Hsu C, et al. Nasal base reduction: a treatment algorithm including alar release with medialization. Plast Reconstr Surg 2009;123(2):716–25.)

usually covered with an antibiotic ointment. Clear ointments such as ophthalmic gentamicin provide a relatively clear view of the wound during the postoperative period. Sutures are usually removed on the fifth to seventh day after the operation.

COMPLICATIONS OF ALAR BASE SURGERY
Visible Scar

Maximum effort is usually made to conceal the scars in normal grooves and shadows of the nose; however, removal of a large piece of tissue, careless excision, and patient susceptibility to scar formation are possible reasons that lead to a visible scar.

Asymmetric Nostrils

Many factors may affect the symmetry of nostrils; however asymmetric alar base resections may result in severe asymmetry. Precise preoperative measurement, excision, and closure is the best known way to avoid this complication.

Notch Formation

Excessive resection and careless closure are the main reasons for nostril notching, which may be easily prevented by a logical treatment plan and precise closure techniques.

Overresection of Nasal Base Tissue

A tendency to make a smaller nose may lead to overresection of nasal tissue. It should be remembered that overresection of soft tissue is extremely difficult to undo, and if any mistake is to happen in the treatment plan it is generally recommended that it be on the side of underresection rather than overresection.

SUMMARY

Nasal base surgery is an extremely sensitive part of rhinoplasty. Diagnosis of nasal base pathology is usually done by clinical examination of the patient and a comprehensive assessment of life-size photographs. Alar flare excess, wide nasal base, and bulky alar tissues are the main problems that are confronted in nasal base surgery. Operative technique is usually designed by preoperative evaluations and intraoperative judgments. If any doubt exists in surgical technique or amount of tissue excision, it is usually recommended that nasal base surgery be postponed for a few weeks to months to allow better evaluation. Visible scar and overresection are the main complications, which may be prevented by a thorough treatment plan and a conservative surgical technique.

SUGGESTED READINGS

Adamson PA, Van Duyne JM. Alar base refinement. Aesthetic Plast Surg 2002;26(Suppl 1):S20.

Becker DG, Weinberger MS, Greene BA, et al. Clinical study of alar anatomy and surgery of the alar base. Arch Otolaryngol Head Neck Surg 1997; 123(8):789–95.

Bennett GH, Lessow A, Song P, et al. The long-term effects of alar base reduction. Arch Facial Plast Surg 2005;7(2):94–7.

Daniel RK. Hispanic rhinoplasty in the United States, with emphasis on the Mexican American nose. Plast Reconstr Surg 2003;112(1):244–56 [discussion: 257–8].

Farkas LG, Hreczko TA, Deutsch CK. Objective assessment of standard nostril types—a morphometric study. Ann Plast Surg 1983;11(5):381–9.

Foda HM. Nasal base narrowing: the combined alar base excision technique. Arch Facial Plast Surg 2007;9(1):30–4.

Gruber R, Kuang A, Khan D. Asian-American rhinoplasty. Aesthet Surg J 2004;24(5):423–30.

Gruber RP, Freeman MB, Hsu C, et al. Nasal base reduction by alar release: a laboratory evaluation. Plast Reconstr Surg 2009;123(2):709–15.

Gruber RP, Freeman MB, Hsu C, et al. Nasal base reduction: a treatment algorithm including alar release with medialization. Plast Reconstr Surg 2009;123 (2):716–25.

Guyuron B. Footplates of the medial crura. Plast Reconstr Surg 1998;101(5):1359–63.

Howley C, Ali N, Lee R, et al. Use of the alar base cinch suture in Le Fort I osteotomy: is it effective? Br J Oral Maxillofac Surg 2011;49(2):127–30.

Kridel RW, Castellano RD. A simplified approach to alar base reduction: a review of 124 patients over 20 years. Arch Facial Plast Surg 2005;7(2):81–93.

Matarasso A. Alar rim excision: a method of thinning bulky nostrils. Plast Reconstr Surg 1996;97(4): 828–34 [discussion: 835].

Millard DR Jr. The alar cinch in the flat, flaring nose. Plast Reconstr Surg 1980;65(5):669–72.

Muradin MS, Rosenberg A, van der Bilt A, et al. The effect of alar cinch sutures and V-Y closure on soft tissue dynamics after Le Fort I intrusion osteotomies. J Craniomaxillofac Surg 2009;37(6): 334–40.

Porter JP, Olson KL. Analysis of the African American female nose. Plast Reconstr Surg 2003;111(2): 620–6 [discussion: 627–8].

Rauso R, Gherardini G, Santillo V, et al. Comparison of two techniques of cinch suturing to avoid widening of the base of the nose after Le Fort I osteotomy. Br J Oral Maxillofac Surg 2010;48(5):356–9.

Rohrich RJ, Ghavami A. Rhinoplasty for Middle Eastern noses. Plast Reconstr Surg 2009;123(4):1343–54.

Rohrich RJ, Hoxworth RE, Thornton JF, et al. The pyriform ligament. Plast Reconstr Surg 2008;121(1): 277–81.

Rohrich RJ, Muzaffar AR. Rhinoplasty in the African-American patient. Plast Reconstr Surg 2003; 111(3):1322–39 [discussion: 1340–1].

Silver WE, Sajjadian A. Nasal base surgery. Otolaryngol Clin North Am 1999;32(4):653–68.

Willis AE 2nd, Costa LE 2nd. Surgical management of the alar base. Atlas Oral Maxillofac Surg Clin North Am 1995;3(2):65–77.

Correction of the Crooked Nose

Jason K. Potter, MD, DDS

KEYWORDS

- Deviated nose • Preoperative assessment
- Intraoperative aspects • Postoperative aspects

Correction of the deviated nose is one of the most difficult tasks in rhinoplasty surgery and should be approached in a systematic manner to ensure a satisfied patient and surgeon. Correction of the deviated nose is unique in that the patient's complaints frequently include aesthetic as well as functional characteristics. Equal importance should be given to the preoperative, intraoperative, and postoperative aspects of the patient's treatment to ensure a favorable outcome.[1,2]

PREOPERATIVE ASSESSMENT

The preoperative assessment includes a comprehensive nasal history, detailed examination of the external and internal nasal structures, documentation of any deformities, establishment of the patient's surgical goals and expectations, and reconciliation of the patient's expectations with the defined deformity. Careful attention to each of these details is essential.

High-quality standardized photographs are an essential part of the preoperative assessment. Photographs allow for documentation and visual explanation of the deformity as well as the goals of the planned procedure. A detailed printed information packet describing the entire perioperative course as well as preoperative and postoperative instructions should be given to every patient at the completion of the initial visit to reinforce the information presented during the consultation. The importance of providing visual and written reinforcement of the preoperative discussion cannot be underestimated.

The initial consultation should achieve 2 main objectives. First, it should provide the surgeon with the opportunity to collect the data that are essential for diagnosis, treatment planning, and performance of the surgical procedure. This is achieved through a systematic and detailed history and physical examination. Second, it should establish a line of communication between the patient and the surgeon to determine if the patient is an appropriate candidate for surgical correction of their deformity. Failure to identify unrealistic expectations, and therefore poor candidates, early will potentially lead to significant problems later. The surgeon should not be afraid to say no to a rhinoplasty patient and decline an operation. An honest and objective surgeon will best inform the patient with realistic expectations.

History

The history should identify the potential cause of the deviated nose (congenital or acquired). It should also establish whether the patient is emotionally, medically, and physically prepared to undergo rhinoplasty. A complete and accurate history identifies the patient's primary concerns (aesthetic and functional), past medical history and review of symptoms, and past surgical history (nasal and other). An appropriate history will identify nasal symptoms, nasal trauma, and current medications. For the deviated nose, it should also identify how and when the deformity occurred.

Special attention should be given to the patient's chief complaint. The specific reason that brought the patient to the office should be documented in the chart. Patients with multiple complaints regarding their nasal appearance should be asked to rank them in order of their objection. It is helpful to have the patient identify the specific concerns while looking at themselves in a handheld mirror to help prevent vague descriptions or explanations that create the

Private Practice, Plastic Surgery, 8220 Walnut Hill Lane, Suite 206, Dallas, TX 75231, USA
E-mail address: potterjason@verizon.net

Oral Maxillofacial Surg Clin N Am 24 (2012) 95–107
doi:10.1016/j.coms.2011.11.001
1042-3699/12/$ – see front matter © 2012 Published by Elsevier Inc.

potential for misunderstanding of the patients expectations. Verbal descriptions of the patient's complaint that are not consistent with their self-identified deformity and physical examination are a clear indication of unrealistic expectations.

Review of the patient's past medical history provides important information to determine a patient's candidacy for surgery. Medical contraindications to rhinoplasty or the need for preoperative medical consultation before surgery should be identified and discussed openly. A patient's overall past surgical history helps to confirm or expand the medical history. Thorough review of any previous nasal surgery or trauma is extremely important at this time. It provides a unique opportunity for the surgeon to gain insight into potential difficulties at the time of surgery. Previous nasal trauma or nasal operations suggest potential structural abnormalities such as septal fracture or surgical absence of local graft material that should be considered in the treatment planning process.

Nasal and upper respiratory symptoms or complaints should be thoroughly investigated and are frequently associated with the deviated nose. These symptoms are usually related to some anatomic deformity or abnormality such as septal deviation, dysfunction of the internal and/or external valves, hypertrophied inferior turbinates, and/or synechiae. Hypertrophied inferior turbinates are often associated with a long history of allergic rhinitis.[3] Such patients must be told that their symptoms of allergic rhinitis may persist for a long time, may not resolve with surgery, and may even be exacerbated during the postoperative period. Patients with a previous history of nasal surgery may have obstruction secondary to synechiae involving the internal structures of the nose, which can recur following correction.

Physical Examination

The anatomic basis of the deviated nose may be related to deformity of the bony pyramid, septal deformation, or a combination of both.[4–9] The physical examination identifies the specific anatomic deformity. This information used in conjunction with the patient's complaints to determine if the patient's goals and expectations are realistic. A systematic detailed examination provides the surgeon with a problem list and foundation from which to form the operative plan. Critical components of the physical examination include facial analysis; surface examination of the dorsum, lobule, and ala; internal nasal examination (with speculum); and assessment of the nasal airflow.

Examination should begin with a full facial analysis (discussed elsewhere in this issue) to assess facial balance and asymmetries as well as identify the potential benefit of adjunctive procedures. Surface characteristics are inspected carefully. Skin thickness and texture, nasal deviation, shape and width, alar rim morphology, tip definition, projection and rotation, nasal base width, and nostril shape should be thoroughly analyzed and documented.

The internal nasal examination begins with a speculum examination to assess the status of the nasal septum and turbinates. It includes assessment of nasal airflow, which is elicited by dynamic maneuvers such as the Cottle test and the use of topical vasoconstrictors. Assessing and documenting the preoperative status of the functional airway is critical to the discussion of potential strategies for surgical improvement of airflow and the interplay these maneuvers have with correction of the external deformity or appearance (spreader grafts and dorsal width). Preexisting septal deformities, perforations, and synechiae should be reported to the patient preoperatively to avoid erroneous blame later. Assessment of cartilage donor sites (especially in patients with a history of trauma and prior nasal surgery) is made when necessary to allow preoperative discussion and justification of distant graft sites (see elsewhere in this issue for complete details of the nasal examination).

THE DEVIATED NOSE

By definition, in the crooked or deviated nose the long axis deviates from the straight vertical orientation of the face.[8,9] Deviation is produced through changes in the osseocartilaginous vault that alter its relationship with the axis of the face. The osseocartilaginous vault should be considered as a dynamic unit because changes to one aspect of this structure can cause alterations to other components. Three basic types of nasal deviation have been described[10] (**Box 1**): caudal septal deviation; concave deformity; concave/convex deformity. The type of deformity should be identified and documented during the nasal examination.

The concave deformity is the most common type of nasal deviation.[10] It may be classified as either C-shaped (left-sided concavity creating a "C" appearance of the nasal dorsum) or reverse C-shaped (right-sided concavity). Concave/convex deformities are the least common and are characterized by deviation of the bony pyramid as well as the septum, which creates an S-shaped appearance of the nose. They are also the most difficult to correct. Caudal septal deviations effect

---

Box 1
Types of nasal deviation

Type I: Caudal septal deviation

> Type Ia: Straight septal tilt. Straight septal tilt off vomer without dorsal septal curvature. Pushes nasal tip off midline. No deviation of nasal pyramid.

> Type Ib: C-shaped septal tilt. Similar to subtype Ia but characterized by C-shaped curvature of caudal septum.

> Type Ic: S-shaped septal tilt. Similar to type Ia but characterized by S-shaped curvature of caudal septum.

Type II: Concave deformity

> Type IIa: C-shaped dorsal deformity: left-sided concavity

> Type IIb: Reverse C-shaped dorsal deformity: right-sided concavity

Type III: Concave/convex. Usually demonstrates both caudal septal deviation and bony pyramid deviation creating an S-shaped dorsal deformity.

Data from Rohrich RJ, Gunter JP, Dueber MA, et al. The deviated nose: optimizing results using a simplified classification and algorithmic approach. Plast Reconstr Surg 2002;110(6):1509–23.

---

changes to the anteroinferior portion of the external nares and can therefore be associated with significant airway compromise.[11]

Deviation of the nasal dorsum can be created by both intrinsic and extrinsic forces acting on the osseocartilaginous vault.[9] Extrinsic forces are those secondary to deviation of the nasal pyramid. These may include forces acting through attachments of the upper and lower cartilages, from deviation of the vomer, perpendicular plate, or maxillary crest. Intrinsic forces are those related to growth of the septal cartilage or deformity of the septal cartilage itself. Correction of nasal deviation requires identification of the cause in each case and appropriate correction. Release of extrinsic forces may allow for correction of the septal or cartilaginous deformity but failure to do so can lead to recurrence.[9] Correction of intrinsic forces requires weakening of the septal cartilage directly or use of suture or grafting techniques that overcome these forces and maintain the desired shape (**Fig. 1**).

Principles of Treatment

Principles of treatment of the crooked nose have been outlined by Byrd and Rohrich (**Box 2**).[9,10]

Key elements of surgical correction include wide exposure to visualize the deformity, release of all extrinsic and intrinsic forces causing the deformity, and reconstruction of the support structures of the nose for longevity of the repair. A useful algorithm incorporating these elements for correction has been described by Rohrich and colleagues[10] and is summarized here. Surgical correction of the deviated nose is based on the following 6 principles: exposure of all deviated structures through an open rhinoplasty approach; release of all septal mucoperichondrial attachments; straightening of the septum; buttressing of septal support with cartilage grafts; reduction or correction of turbinate deformities as necessary to allow for correction of deviated septum; and precise nasal osteotomies.

Surgical Exposure

An open rhinoplasty approach is the preferred method for surgical exposure of deviated nasal structures. It has been demonstrated to provide improved exposure, visualization, and surgical control compared with closed rhinoplasty techniques. The open approach also facilitates wide release of all attachments to the deviated structures. Exposure is created by a transcolumellar and infracartilaginous incision with careful wide elevation of the skin envelope over the nasal dorsum.

Release of Mucoperichondrial Attachments

Extrinsic deforming forces act through the attachments of the upper and lower cartilages and mucoperiosteum of the septum. Through these attachments, they may also affect changes to the nasal tip. Mucoperichondrial attachments to all deviated portions of the nasal septum must be released. This is performed by wide subperichondrial undermining of the septal mucosa on each side of the nasal septum. Exposure of the vomerine septum allows for correction of vomer deformities that may be contributing to nasal airflow obstruction. Mucoperichondrial release may be performed through a separate septal mucosal incision (Keen approach) or by approaching the septum dorsally through the open approach. The dorsal approach facilitates release of the upper lateral cartilages from the septum, improved visualization of the septal deformity and its correction, as well as placement of spreader grafts later in the operation (**Fig. 2**). The upper lateral cartilages are further separated from the lower lateral cartilages at the scroll area and the lower lateral cartilages are released from the maxillary crest as needed.

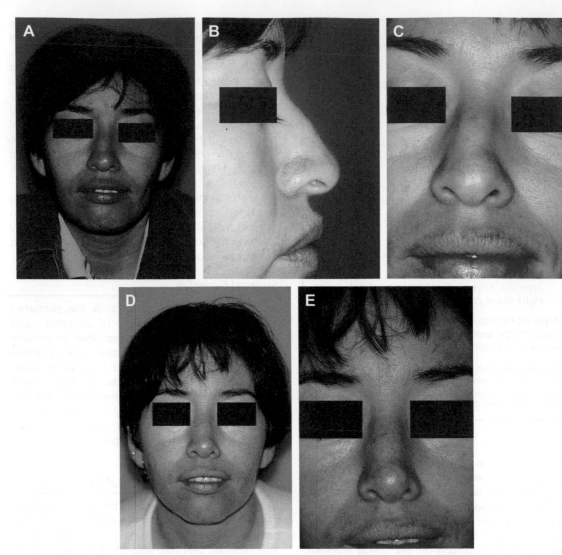

Fig. 1. (A–C) A 32-year-old woman presented for rhinoplasty. The procedure included dorsal reduction, cephalic trim, submucous septal resection, and placement of a caudal strut. (A–C) Preoperative. (D–E) Postoperative. Note recurrent dorsal deflection that could likely have been corrected with unilateral spreader grafts to overpower intrinsic septal forces.

Straightening of the Septum

After release of all extrinsic forces on the septum, it should be inspected for persistent deformity. Persistent deformity is usually secondary to intrinsic forces and must be corrected. Submucous resection of the septum is the preferred approach. The area of the deformity is resected under direct visualization taking care to maintain a 1-cm dorsal and caudal L-strut for long-term structural integrity (**Fig. 3**). It is extremely important to maintain the integrity of the septum with the nasal bones superiorly for dorsal nasal support. If the septum is deviated from the midline at its attachment at the maxillary crest, this may be released, moved to the midline and resecured

with permanent suture (**Fig. 4**). Deviations isolated to the inferocaudal septum may be corrected with a swing door septal flap. This is created through a vertical wedge resection of the septal cartilage on the convex side at the point of caudal deviation (**Fig. 5**). Any persistent warping of the cartilage present after these maneuvers should be addressed through cartilage scoring to interrupt the cartilage memory and reinforced with cartilage grafting to maintain the desired position.

Buttressing Septal Support

Septal support is critical for dorsal nasal relationships of the midvault of the nose. It should therefore be reinforced after septal surgery. Spreader

Box 2
Principles of correction of the deviated nose

1. Exposure of all deviated structures through an open rhinoplasty approach

2. Release of all septal mucoperichondrial attachments

3. Straightening of the septum

4. Buttressing of septal support with cartilage grafts

5. Reduction or correction of turbinate deformities as necessary to allow for correction of the deviated septum

6. Precise nasal osteotomies

Data from Rohrich RJ, Gunter JP, Dueber MA, et al. The deviated nose: optimizing results using a simplified classification and algorithmic approach. Plast Reconstr Surg 2002;110(6):1509–23.

grafts are ideal for maintaining the long-term integrity of the weakened dorsal septal cartilage (**Fig. 6**).[12] These grafts are ideally fashioned from the cartilage harvested during the submucous resection. They are fashioned 5–6 mm in height and should extend the length of the dorsal septum. It is important to recognize that placement of spreader grafts can potentially widen the appearance of the nasal dorsum. In situations where this is objectionable to the aesthetic outcome, they should be positioned several millimeters inferior to the dorsal edge of the septum to minimize this effect.[13] In situations of persistent concave deformity, this effect may be used to correct the

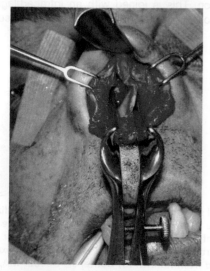

Fig. 2. Exposure of septal deformity through the dorsal approach to septal cartilage.

concavity by unilateral placement on the concave side. The grafts are secured with two 5-0 clear nylon sutures. Additional grafting to strengthen the caudal portion of the septum and provide tip support may be necessary. This is achieved with placement of a caudal strut between the middle crura of the lower lateral cartilages.

Reduction of Hypertrophied Turbinates

Evaluation of the size and position of the inferior turbinate is an important component of management of the deviated nose. Septal deviation is often associated with contralateral inferior turbinate hypertrophy. Reduction of the inferior turbinate is important if it impedes repositioning the septum to the midline, is associated with preoperative nasal airflow obstruction, or its persistence would lead to nasal airflow obstruction after repositioning the septum (creates critical airway narrowing). Reduction is performed with a submucosal resection of the turbinate.[14]

Nasal Osteotomies

Deformity of the bony pyramid is a frequent component of the deviated nose. Extrinsic deforming forces on the septum may be created by this deformity. Occasionally, the bony deviation and septal deviation may be in opposite directions and in this situation, correction of the bony deviation may magnify the septal deformity.[9] Byrd (**Box 3**) has classified the bony deformity into 3 categories: a symmetric pyramid that is deviated from the aesthetic midline of the face; a deviated pyramid with a prominent nasal dorsum; and a deviated bony pyramid with asymmetry of the nasal bones. Precise osteotomies are required for correction of all 3 categories. Osteotomies may be performed through internal or external approaches and using a perforated or continuous technique. Percutaneous, lateral, perforated osteotomies have the advantage of precise control, minimal bruising and swelling, and less likelihood of disruption of the nasal mucosa.[15] Percutaneous osteotomies are performed with a sharp 2-mm osteotome near the junction of the nasal sidewall with the frontal process of the maxilla. Care must be taken to avoid the angular branch of the facial vessel to minimize bruising. Type I deformities are corrected through lateral osteotomies of nasal bones and greenstick fracture of the perpendicular plate of the ethmoid bone that allow for movement of a symmetric nasal pyramid to the aesthetic facial midline. Dorsal reduction is not necessary (**Fig. 7**A). Type II deformities require resection of the prominent nasal dorsum initially. Lateral percutaneous osteotomies are then performed to allow

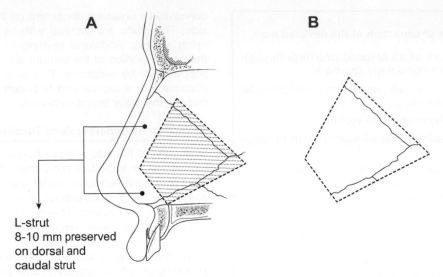

A

B

L-strut
8-10 mm preserved
on dorsal and
caudal strut

Fig. 3. (*A*) 1-cm dorsal and caudal strut should be maintained after submucous resection of the septum. (*B*) Osseocartilaginous septal specimen resected.

correction of the osseous deformity. The open-roof deformity created during resection of the prominent dorsum provides separation of the nasal bones allowing their independent correction (see **Fig. 7**B). Type III deformities require both medial and lateral nasal osteotomies for correction (see **Fig. 7**C). This combination frees the nasal bones from the frontal process of the maxilla as well as from each other to create the opportunity for independent movement of the nasal bones and correction of the asymmetric deformity.[9]

Sequencing Treatment

The procedure begins with surgical preparation of the nose. Internal nasal vibrissae are trimmed

with fine scissors to improve visualization. Local anesthesia is infiltrated into the septal mucosa bilaterally and the dorsal nasal soft tissues with several milliliters of local anesthetic with epineph-rine solution (**Fig. 8**). Care should be taken to minimize the volume injected to prevent excessive distortion and thickness of the soft tissue envelope during the procedure. The nasal airways are then prepped with betadine or other appropriate solution and the nasal vault is packed bilaterally with several pledgets soaked in oxymetolazone. The remainder of the face is then sterilely prepped.

The incision begins at the narrowest portion of the columella with a stair-stepped transcolumellar incision. This is joined with an infracartilaginous incision within each naris. Sharp scissor dissection

A

B

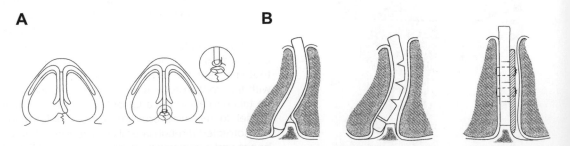

Fig. 4. (*A–B*) Techniques for correcting a deflected inferocaudal septum at the maxillary crest. (*A*) Mobilization and secured with permanent suture. (*B*) Mobilization, cartilage scoring, and stabilization with cartilage graft. The curved septum is straightened by removing small wedges of cartilage from the convex side. Inferior septal excision in the vomerine groove is often needed. A batten cartilage graft is secured with 5-0 polydioxanone mattress sutures to stabilize the straightened septum. (*Adapted from* Rohrich RJ, Gunter JP, Dueber MA, et al. The deviated nose: optimizing results using a simplified classification and algorithmic approach. Plast Reconstr Surg 2002;110(6):1509–23.)

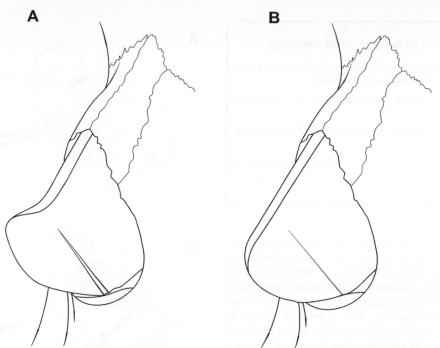

Fig. 5. Septal swing door flap for correction of a curvature deformity of the inferocaudal septum. (*A*) A swinging door flap is used to straighten the deviated, but not curved, caudal septum. (*B*) The swinging door flap is sutured securely to the periosteum of the nasal spine. (*Adapted from* Rohrich RJ, Gunter JP, Dueber MA, et al. The deviated nose: optimizing results using a simplified classification and algorithmic approach. Plast Reconstr Surg 2002;110(6):1509–23.)

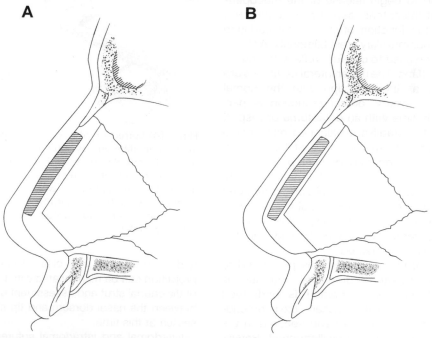

Fig. 6. Spreader graft placement. Spreader grafts are secured to the dorsal septal strut. They may be placed at the dorsal edge of the septal cartage if dorsal widening is desired or may be placed inferior to the dorsal edge to mitigate their effect on dorsal widening. (*A*) Spreader grafts may be placed invisibly, above the dorsal septal plane; or visibly, at or below the dorsal septal plane (*B*) either to widen the midvault or to elevate the dorsum. Unilateral placement may be used to camouflage any residual dorsal curvature. (*Adapted from* Rohrich RJ, Gunter JP, Dueber MA, et al. The deviated nose: optimizing results using a simplified classification and algorithmic approach. Plast Reconstr Surg 2002;110(6):1509–23.)

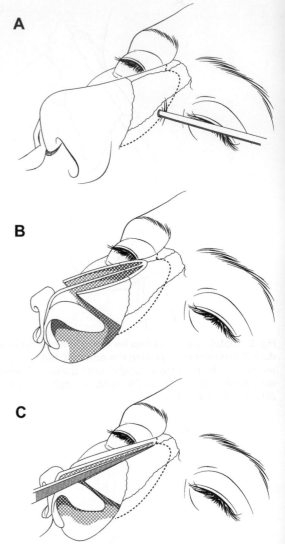

is then used to separate the overlying subcutaneous tissue from the alar cartilages in the supraperichondrial plane. Dissection continues over the upper lateral cartilages onto the nasal bones. Over the nasal bones, the plane of dissection is transitioned subperiosteally. The extent of deformity can now be assessed. The attachment of the lower lateral cartilages with the upper lateral cartilages is released though a modest cephalic trim. Care should be taken to maintain a minimum width of 6–8 mm of the lateral crura to optimize its structural integrity.

The septum is then approached dorsally. A 15 blade is used to begin release of the mucoperichondrium at the anterior septal angle continuing inferiorly to the junction of the septal cartilage with the anterior maxillary crest bilaterally. A Cottle elevator is then used to carefully reflect the mucoperichondrial flaps. The upper lateral cartilages are then incised at their junction with the dorsal septum. If necessary, dorsal reduction is performed at this time with an osteotome or rasp. It is important to establish a balanced relationship of the dorsum with the nasal tip at this time. If asymmetric nasal bones are present, proper orientation of the reduction is critical. In this situation, the more vertically oriented nasal bone is reduced less so that a symmetric bone height is achieved after correction of the nasal bone position with osteotomies. Osteotomies are performed and the dorsal deviation is corrected.

Inspection of the septum is now performed to reassess the extent of deformity. Submucous resection of the central portion is performed leaving a 1-cm L-strut. If necessary, the inferocaudal septum can be released and secured in the midline at the level of the maxillary crest. Persistent intrinsic deformities of the septum are corrected with cartilage scoring.

Spreader and columellar strut grafts are then fashioned from the previously harvested septal cartilage. These are then positioned appropriately

Fig. 7. (*A*) Correction of a type I bony deformity with lateral percutaneous osteotomies. (*B*) Correction of a type II bony deformity with dorsal reduction and lateral percutaneous osteotomies. (*C*) Correction of a type III bony deformity with medial and lateral osteotomies. (*Data from* Byrd HS, Salomon J, Flood J. Correction of the crooked nose. Plast Reconstr Surg 1998;102:2148.)

and secured with 5-0 clear nylon suture. Tip projection can be manipulated with the placement of the caudal strut and assessment of the balance between the nasal dorsum and tip should be assessed at this time.

Interdomal and intradomal sutures are placed for tip refinement as appropriate. The wound is irrigated copiously and attention is turned toward closure. The nasal soft tissues are redraped and the ideal profile and dorsal aesthetic lines are assessed. Closure is performed with 6-0 nylon at

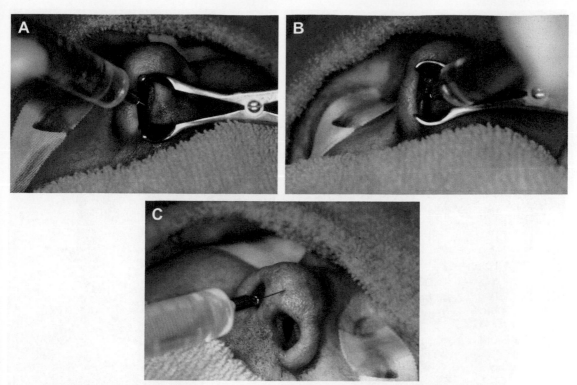

Fig. 8. (*A*) Injection of the septal mucosa. (*B*) Injection of the plane of dissection for infracartilaginous incision. (*C*) Injection of dorsal soft tissues.

the transcolumellar incision and percutaneous osteotomy sites and 4-0 chromic for repair of the infracartilaginous incision. Doyle splints are placed with copious antibiotic ointment and secured at the membranous septum with a 3-0 silk suture. Taping of the nasal dorsum is performed to redrape the soft tissues intimately with the newly established osseocartilaginous framework (**Fig. 9**). Taping is begun at the level of the supratip break. An external nasal splint is applied.

CASE EXAMPLE

A 19-year-old woman presented for correction of her deviated nasal deformity (**Fig. 10**). Her chief complaint pertained to the deviated nose and difficulty breathing through the right naris. She had a history of right unilateral cleft lip and palate. Past medical history was otherwise unremarkable. Past surgical history was significant for primary lip and palate repair as a child and secondary revision of her cheiloplasty as an adolescent. She denied previous nasal surgery but did report difficulty breathing through the right naris. On physical examination she demonstrated an S-shaped dorsal deformity, slight dorsal prominence, down-turned nasal tip with hypertrophic lip scarring, poor tip defining points, septal

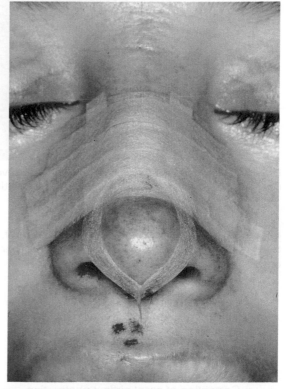

Fig. 9. Taping of soft tissues to facilitate adaption to the osseocartilaginous skeleton.

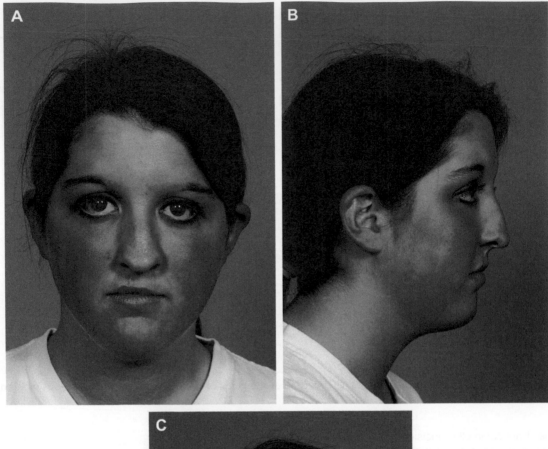

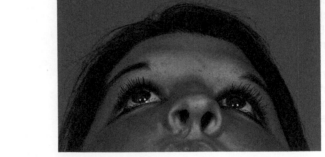

Fig. 10. (*A–C*) A 19-year-old woman with preoperative deviated nasal deformity. (*A*) Preoperative anterioposterior view. (*B*) Preoperative lateral view. (*C*) Preoperative worm's eye view.

deviation, and a positive Cottle test on the right. She also demonstrated a malalignment of her cupids bow.

The operative goals included (**Fig. 11**):

- Correction of dorsal deviation and reestablishing aesthetic dorsal lines
- Reduction of the dorsal hump
- Improved tip projection
- Refining the tip definition
- Correction of the septal deformity
- Correction of nasal airflow obstruction
- Improvement of the cleft lip deformity

The surgical treatment plan consisted of:

- Open rhinoplasty approach
- Osseous and cartilaginous dorsal reduction
- Percutaneous lateral nasal osteotomies
- Correction of septal deviation with submucous resection
- Septal reconstruction with spreader grafts and caudal strut secured with intercrural sutures
- Refinement of the nasal tip with cephalic trim and transdomal and intradomal suture techniques

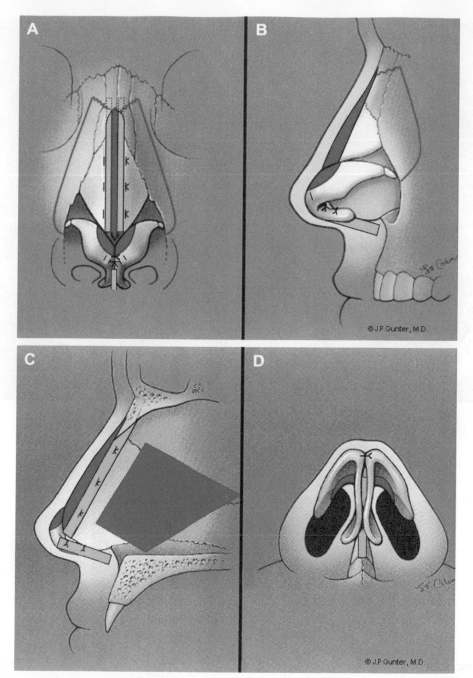

Fig. 11. Gunter graphic demonstrating the surgical maneuvers performed (*A–D*). (*A*) Percutaneous lateral nasal osteotomies, spreader grafts, cephalic trim. (*B*) Dorsal nasal reduction, percutaneous lateral nasal osteotomies, cephalic trim, and caudal strut. (*C*) Spreader graft placement and submucous resection. (*D*) Tip refinement with suturing techniques. (*Courtesy of* J.P. Gunter, MD, Dallas, TX.)

- Correction of nasal airflow obstruction with correction of septal deviation and spreader grafts
- Revision of cleft lip deformity

The patient is shown approximately 9 months postoperatively (**Fig. 12**). Note the straight nasal dorsum and improved dorsal aesthetic lines. Nasal projection and tip definition are improved. The lateral view demonstrates improved dorsal balance between the osseocartilaginous vault and nasal tip as a result of the dorsal reduction and improved tip projection. She also demonstrated improved appearance of the nasolabial

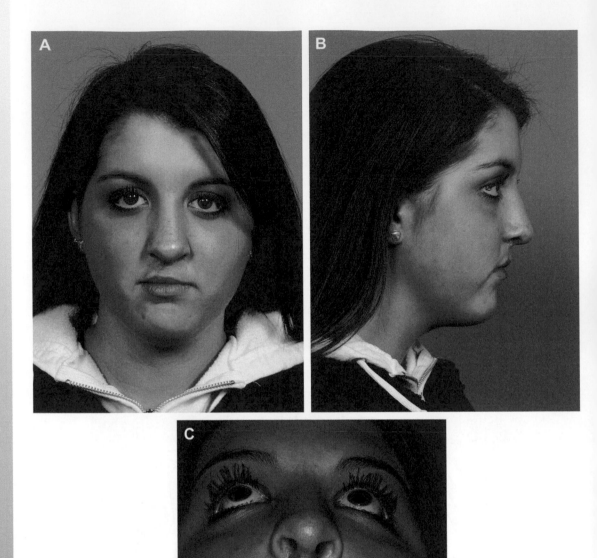

Fig. 12. (*A–C*) Results 9 months after surgery. (*A*) Postoperative anterioposterior view. (*B*) Postoperative lateral view. (*C*) Postoperative worm's eye view.

relationships secondary to revision of her cleft lip deformity. The worm's eye demonstrates improvement in her intranasal septal deformity, alar base relationships, and cleft lip deformity.

REFERENCES

1. Rohrich RJ. Rhinoplasty planning. Dallas Rhinoplasty Symp 1995;12:67.
2. Rohrich RJ, Byrd HS, Oneal RM, et al. Management of the rhinoplasty patient.
3. Courtiss EH, Gargan TJ, Courtiss GB. Nasal physiology. Ann Plast Surg 1984;13:214.
4. Dingman RO, Natvig P. The deviated nose. Clin Plast Surg 1977;4:145.
5. Johnson CM, Anderson JR. The deviated nose: its correction. Laryngoscope 1977;87:1680.
6. Mckinney P, Shively R. Straightening the twisted nose. Plast Reconstr Surg 1979;64:176.
7. Brian DF. The management of the deviated nose. J Laryngol Otol 1981;95:471.
8. Gunter JP, Rohrich RJ. Management of the deviated nose. The importance of septal reconstruction. Clin Plast Surg 1988;15(1):43.
9. Byrd HS, Salomon J, Flood J. Correction of the crooked nose. Plast Reconstr Surg 1998;102:2148.

10. Rohrich RJ, Gunter JP, Dueber MA, et al. The deviated nose: optimizing results using a simplified classification and algorithmic approach. Plast Reconstr Surg 2002;110(6):1509.

11. Guyuron B, Uzzo CD, Scull H. A practical classification of septonasal deviation and an effective guide to septal surgery. Plast Reconstr Surg 1999;104: 2202.

12. Sheen JH. Spreader grafts: a method of reconstructing the roof of the middle nasal vault following rhinoplasty. Plast Reconstr Surg 1984;73:230.

13. Rohrich RJ, Hollier LH. Use of spreader grafts in the external approach to rhinoplasty. Clin Plast Surg 1996;23:255.

14. Rohrich RJ, Krueger JK, Adams WP, et al. Rationale for submucous resection of the hypertrophied inferior turbinates in rhinoplasty: an evolution. Plast Reconstr Surg 2001;108(2):536.

15. Rohrich RJ, Minoli JJ, Adams WP, et al. The lateral nasal osteotomy in rhinoplasty: an anatomic endoscopic comparison of the external versus internal approach. Plast Reconstr Surg 1997;99:1309.

Internal Septorhinoplasty Technique

Peter D. Waite, MPH, DDS, MD

KEYWORDS

- Internal septorhinoplasty • Endonasal technique
- Internal rhinoplasty • Cosmetic surgery

The internal septorhinoplasty, also known as the closed nasal or endonasal technique, was the standard operating procedure until the popularity of the external or open rhinoplasty technique. The advantages of the internal technique are several (**Box 1**). Patient satisfaction is better, especially for the experienced surgeon. For specific changes in nasal configuration, the internal rhinoplasty can be used with specificity. In fact, all of the same surgical manipulations can be performed through an internal rhinoplasty as in an external rhinoplasty.[1] Patient satisfaction is usually better because there is no scar across the columella, less edema, and a quicker recovery. The addition of a transcolumella scar may produce decreased lymphatic drainage. The internal approach is more predictable because the skin drape can be easily analyzed and the surgeon can quickly assess the cosmetic changes attributable to the cartilage reduction. Unless extensive tip grafting and cartilage augmentation is performed, the internal approach is usually a faster technique, with quicker dissection and closure.[2,3] External skin sutures are not required. For patients that require simple hump reduction or nasal narrowing, the internal approach is simplistic and allows simultaneous septoplasty (**Fig. 1**). It is important for the cosmetic surgeon to realize the enemy of good is better. Oftentimes striving to overachieve can only result in disastrous results. A simple internal rhinoplasty will produce a very good result and satisfied patients.

Surgical time and efficiency in all procedures is important. Certainly, hastily performed surgical procedures will yield poor results. On the other hand, surgeons that seem to dawdle and lose perspective with extensive operating time also experience diminished results. Therefore, simple tried-and-true surgical techniques, such as internal rhinoplasty, when used with a specific, focused treatment plan based on a solid diagnosis, will yield excellent results.

The disadvantage of the internal rhinoplasty is primarily the fact that it is a difficult concept for the novice to understand and perform (**Box 2**). It is difficult for the beginner to visualize the internal incisions and understand the relationship of the nasal cartilage. Therefore, the external rhinoplasty is a good technique for the novice but may not always be necessary as the surgeon develops experience. Certainly, dorsal hump reduction without a tip rhinoplasty is very amenable to internal rhinoplasty techniques.[3] Patients with complex deformities, such as revision rhinoplasty, cleft noses, and twisted tip deformities following complex trauma, may be better suited for the external rhinoplasty technique.[1] Also, extensive tip-grafting techniques are difficult to secure via the internal technique. Shield grafts, tip grafts, and other such cartilage grafting to the tip of the nose can be performed much more precisely and easily secured through an external technique, but these same procedures can also be done by experienced surgeons through an internal technique with good results.[4] It is true that the internal rhinoplasty requires several more precise incisions to properly provide access to the septum, dorsum, and lower lateral cartilages. Therefore, internal

Department of Oral & Maxillofacial Surgery, University of Alabama at Birmingham, Birmingham, AL, USA
E-mail address: pwaite@uab.edu

Oral Maxillofacial Surg Clin N Am 24 (2012) 109–117
doi:10.1016/j.coms.2011.10.008
1042-3699/12/$ – see front matter Published by Elsevier Inc.

rhinoplasty does require precise placement of incisions to prevent unnatural scarring and retraction of the nose.[5]

In rhinoplasty, there are 5 basic nasal surgical steps (**Box 3**). These steps should be closely followed both in the evaluation of the nose and in surgical execution.[1] The surgeon must remember that *airway* is first. The septum must first be carefully evaluated and the deviations identified. Septal deviations left untreated can result in the deviation of the nose. The septal deviation can act as a rudder on a boat and allow the nose to deviate, especially after several fixation points have been released. In septorhinoplasty, the septum should be corrected first. If there is any doubt of airway obstruction or septal deviation, this problem must be addressed. It is important to remember that rhinoplasty often makes the nose smaller and may compromise the nasal valve, which could leave patients with more complaints of airway obstruction after a rhinoplasty if the septoplasty was not performed. Always remember the airway

is number 1, and airflow is a functional medical problem and not a cosmetic problem. Airflow is objective, whereas nasal configuration and shape are subjective and cosmetic.

1. The standard septoplasty can be approached by exposing the caudal edge of the nasal septum. This area is usually accessed through an incomplete transfixion incision when performing an internal septorhinoplasty. Local anesthesia with epinephrine will help provide hemostasis and hydro-dissection (**Figs. 2** and **3**). The intercartilaginous incision will come to join the transfixion incision bilaterally and give access to the dorsum (**Fig. 4**). Working through the right nostril, the caudal edge of the nasal septum is exposed and the perichondrium scored. A #15 blade can be used to lightly make a tic-tac-toe–type incision through the perichondrium (**Fig. 5**). This procedure will allow a dental condenser or caudal elevator to gain access beneath the perichondrium (**Fig. 6**). The perichondrial pocket is then further developed, gaining access to the quadrangular septum and the perpendicular plate to the ethmoid and fulmar. The septal deviation must be identified, and, in most situations, the deviation is excised as in the submucosal resection. A Balanger swivel knife (KLS Martin Corp., Jacksonville, FL, USA) or caudal elevator can be used to sharply cut through the quadrangular septum and carefully elevate the left-side perichondrium. Usually, the quadrangular septum is disarticulated from the perpendicular

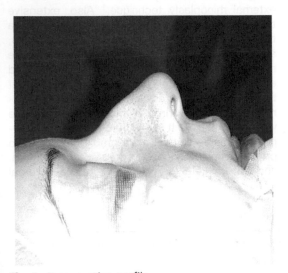

Fig. 1. Preoperative profile.

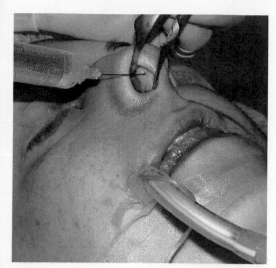

Fig. 2. Local anesthesia injected into the membranous septum.

plate of the ethmoid and fulmar and released from the nasal maxillary crest (**Fig. 7**). It is important to leave at least 7 to 8 mm of quadrangular septum along the dorsum and

columella to prevent a saddle deformity.[3] After the deviated portion of the septum has been resected, the surgeon must carefully evaluate for perforations and re-approximate the nasal mucosa with a transseptal chromic suture. Silastic nasal stents can be placed at the close of the rhinoplasty.

2. Step 2 is skeletonizing the nose and exposing the dorsal hump. This procedure is done through dissection through the intercartilaginous incision over the upper lateral cartilage onto the nasal bones.[5–7] Some surgeons like to elevate the periosteum, but special care must be maintained to prevent disarticulation of the upper lateral cartilage from the nasal bone. A button knife or scissors can be used to develop this subcutaneous pocket over the dorsum only to the extent of the lateral nasal osteotomy. An Aufricht or Converse (KLS Martin Corp., Jacksonville, FL, USA) nasal retractor usually works well to retract the dorsal skin and give access to the bony and cartilaginous hump (**Fig. 8**A). The retractor will also protect the skin from the surgeon's knife while reducing the dorsal hump. The surgeon can then use a #15 blade or #11 blade to

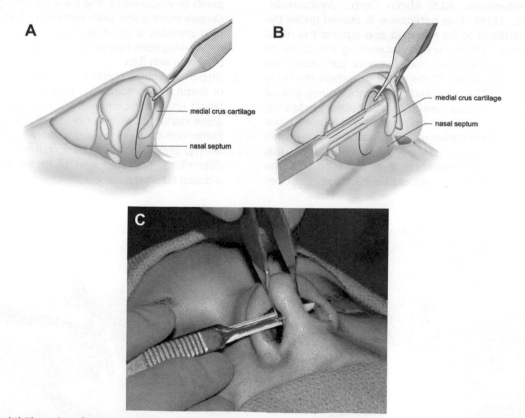

Fig. 3. (A) The Adson forceps retracting and protecting the medial crural cartilage. (B) The knife blade stops short of cutting through the medial crural footplate that overlaps the septum and supports the tip. (C) Incomplete transfixion incision through the membranous septum exposing the caudal edge of the septum.

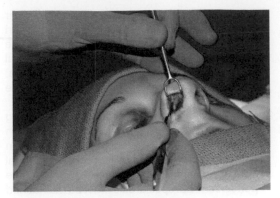

Fig. 4. Intercartilaginous incision.

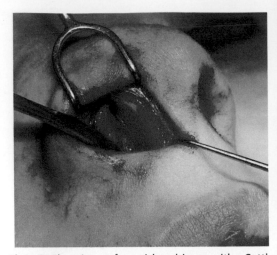

Fig. 6. Elevation of perichondrium with Cottle elevator (KLS Martin, Jacksonville, FL, USA).

horizontally reduce the cartilaginous hump extending from the rhinion to the superior septal angle. A common mistake at this point is to leave cartilage in the area of the supratip break, which will ultimately lead to a poly beak deformity. The amount of cartilage excised is an artistic decision and based on clinical experience (see **Fig. 8**B). The dorsal hump is then further reduced by the introduction of a nasal osteotome or Rubin osteotome (KLS Martin Corp., Jacksonville, FL, USA). This osteotome is placed under the cartilage to be resected and against the nasal bone. While carefully observing the angle of the osteotomy, the surgeon can now use a mallet against the chisel to reduce the bony hump. The bone and cartilaginous hump should be recovered carefully without pulling or tearing mucosa. A common mistake is to remove more bone than cartilage. This practice will also result in a poly beak deformity. As a general rule, this author recommends that two-thirds of the hump resection should be cartilage and one-

third should be bony. After the dorsal hump is removed, this may produce the proper profile but will leave an open roof deformity. Slight irregularities can be corrected with a series of nasal rasps. The surgeon should carefully use a coarse to fine file to reduce any bony, sharp points or irregularities. The bone file will usually remove more bone than cartilage. This time also provides a good opportunity to remove any cartilaginous fragments or bone debris left under the skin flap.

3. Step 3 is the correction of the lateral nasal width or shape. This procedure is performed through lateral nasal osteotomies, which is really, by some standards, still part of step 2, the dorsal hump reduction. However, in some patients with no significant dorsal hump but with lateral deformities, this step can be done without a dorsal hump reduction.[3]

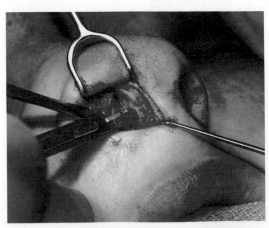

Fig. 5. Crosscut perichondrium aids in elevation.

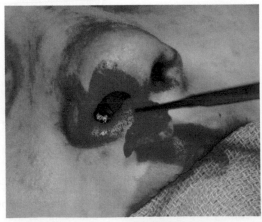

Fig. 7. Caudal deflection of septum.

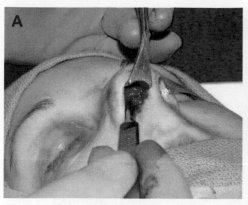
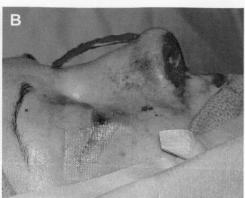

Fig. 8. (*A*) Dorsal exposure with Aufricht retractor. A #15 blade is cutting off the cartilage hump. (*B*) Dorsal hump reduction. Note most of the hump reduction is cartilage.

A nasal speculum is used to cradle the edge of the piriform aperture just at the junction of the inferior turbinate. A #15 blade is used to make a horizontal incision or stab incision along the edge of the piriform rim. A caudal elevator is then used to initiate a submucosal pocket. A straight Nivert chisel (KLS Martin Corp., Jacksonville, FL, USA) is ideal for the lateral nasal osteotomy. The working edge of this osteotomy is only a few millimeters of the sharp corner of the chisel. The guard should be placed externally to prevent tearing the nasal mucosa and adds in digital detection of the proper placement of the osteotomy (**Fig. 9**). The osteotomy need not extend all the way up to the medial canthus. The osteotomy in effect makes a series of perforations in the bone, which allows for the frontal process of the maxilla to collapse medially, thereby reducing the open roof deformity. The lateral osteotomy should be performed on both sides in a symmetric fashion. Beginning the osteotomy too high on the nose may be unesthetic and beginning too low will detach or allow the anterior portion of the inferior turbinate to fall into the nose, thereby causing a functional airway obstruction. This small incision along the nasal aperture never needs primary closure.

4. Step 4: The tip of the nose is addressed next. The delicate artistic refinements of the nasal tip should be done after the more bulky, heavy foundational surgery of the osteotomies. Some surgeons prefer to set the tip before dorsal hump reduction, but this is a matter of surgical preference. Tip rhinoplasty is an article in itself. There are many techniques and procedures to correct tip abnormalities.

It is best to keep it simple on the primary septorhinoplasty and time has proven that overoperation of the nasal tip results in scarring, atrophy, retraction, and an unnatural appearance. The best tip procedure is the preservation of cartilage as in the complete resection.[8] The lateral crural cartilage can be modified best if delivered, which requires the design of a bipedicle flap. The intercartilaginous incision already performed is part of the access to the lower lateral cartilages. The surgeon must create a marginal incision so that the lateral crural cartilage can be delivered as a bucket handle, swiveling from the medial crural footpad and lateral crural footpad. A double skin hook is introduced on the edge of the alar, and a #15 blade can be used to tick or feel the inferior edge of the lateral crural cartilage. A small incision is made, and the side of the #15 blade can provide tactile direction for the incision. The #15 blade is extended from the lateral crural cartilage toward the medial aspect of the nose along the marginal incision into the dome of the nose. Access is difficult, and it is extremely difficult to follow the

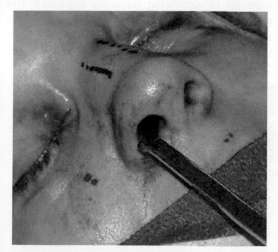

Fig. 9. Lateral nasal osteotomy. The working edge of the Nivert chisel engages the bone, and the guard is palpated under the skin.

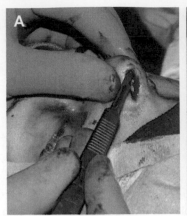
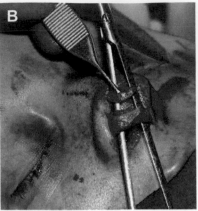

Fig. 10. (*A*) Marginal incision begins at the mucocutaneous junction along the columella. Note the surgeon pinches and twists the tip to gain exposure under the soft triangle. (*B*) The lateral crus is exposed by the cartilage delivery technique. The intercartilaginous and marginal incision allow the lower lateral cartilage to rotate off a bipedicle flap. This procedure demonstrates the complete strip tip rhinoplasty.

crural cartilage without transecting it. Therefore, it is better to make a similar marginal incision on the medial crural cartilage at the mucocutaneous junction. This procedure is done by a maneuver of holding the tip of the nose in the surgeon's left hand between the thumb and index finger with slight rotation. The #15 blade can then be placed into the dome of the nose and an incision created along the mucocutaneous border (**Fig. 10**A). This incision will allow access between the 2 medial crural cartilages, and the marginal incision is simply connected from the lateral aspect medially into the dome of the nose. As the cartilage becomes visible, the dissection must proceed carefully between the cartilage and the skin, staying as close as possible to the cartilage without transection. As the dissection proceeds over the crural cartilage, it will enter into the intercartilaginous incision, which will create a bipedicle flap of the medial and lateral edges of the crural cartilage. The crural cartilage can then be

delivered out of the nostril, and direct access is achieved (see **Fig. 10**B).

A complete strip is named for the amount of cartilage that is left behind.[8] A #15 blade is then used to excise all but about 4 to 5 mm of the lateral crural cartilage. In effect, this resects a portion of the superior edge of the crural cartilage and allows for retraction and volumetric reduction of the tip. When done bilaterally, it will also allow for slight tip rotation. Both the left and right crural cartilages need to be freely released without sacrificing the overlapping ligament of the medial crural footpads. This support mechanism is important in the tripod concept of the nasal tip. The surgeon should always strive to maintain tip projection because almost every incision made in the internal rhinoplasty has the potential of sacrificing nasal tip support.[8] The usual plan is to allow tip rotation and a more youthful appearance without sacrificing nasal projection (**Figs. 11–17**). The nasal tip should be

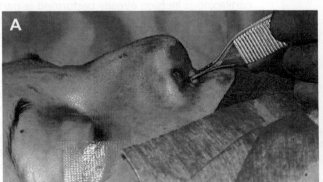
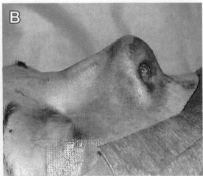

Fig. 11. (*A*) Quick check of supratip break. If nasal projection is lost by lack of tip support, a poly beak deformity may result. (*B*) Profile with good supratip break at surgery.

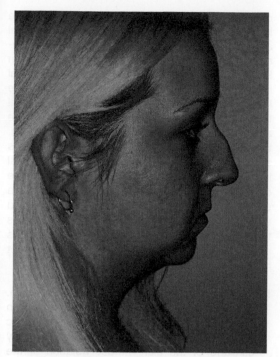

Fig. 12. Preoperative view demonstrates a large dorsal hump easily treated by internal rhinoplasty.

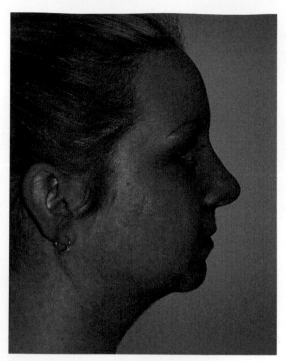

Fig. 14. Postoperative lateral profile.

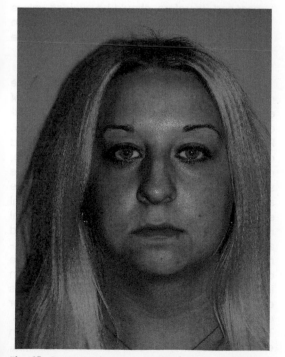

Fig. 13. Preoperative view in the frontal profile.

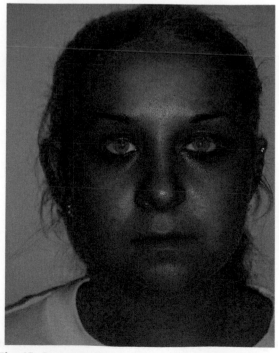

Fig. 15. Postoperative frontal profile.

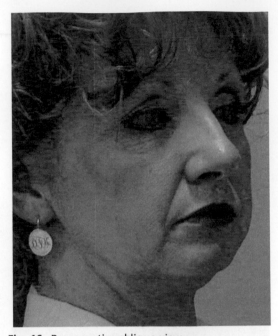

Fig. 16. Preoperative oblique view.

slightly strong and offset with an obvious supratip break at the end of the operation. If the tip of the nose is excessively broad and the intermediate crural cartilage significantly deviated, the cartilages may be divided as in a Goldman tip and the medial sewn together. This procedure will greatly narrow the nose and preserve tip projection. In fact, in some cases, cartilage projection

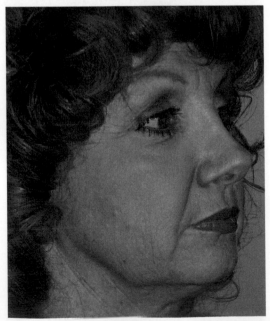

Fig. 17. Two-year postoperative oblique view of internal rhinoplasty with good tip support.

can be increased by stealing cartilage from the lateral and sewing it together to increase a medial as in a medial strut.[9] Failure to perform this accurately and leaving irregularities can result in knuckling or an asymmetric tip. The marginal incision should be carefully closed along the lateral portion of the incision to prevent the lateral footpad of the cartilage from falling into the nose and causing a functional airway obstruction. Usually two 4-0 or 5-0 fast-absorbing gut sutures are placed along the lateral aspect of the marginal incision. One other key stitch is placed in the dome to reposition the cartilage. Correct closure of the marginal incision is very important and should be done symmetrically. If the nose is taped and stented properly, very few incisions are necessary and will usually allow for correct healing.

5. Step 5 is the correction of the nasal base or ala. This procedure is seldom required except in abnormal alar base deformities. The basic Wier procedure is a resection of the fibrofatty cartilage of the alar without violation of the nasal seal, which is sometimes beneficial in Asian and African nasal deformities.[10] Alar resection is also indicated in asymmetrical nasal base deformities, such as cleft lip and palate. It may also be used symmetrically following abnormal flaring of the nasal base in orthognathic surgery. Alar base resections and Wier procedures usually leave a small scar and, therefore, should be avoided unless absolutely necessary. This procedure can always be performed at a secondary procedure under local anesthesia if necessary.

In conclusion, the internal technique of the rhinoplasty should be in the armamentarium of every cosmetic surgeon. There will always be indications for both internal and external rhinoplasty. Rhinoplasty should be treatment planned based on the individual diagnosis. With experience, most surgeons find the internal rhinoplasty to be successful and extremely rewarding. The novice should remember the 5 basic steps of nasal surgery, whether performing internal or external rhinoplasty. The septum is important and should always be considered first. It most likely will determine the functional outcome of the airway.[2] The dorsal hump can easily be accessed through an internal rhinoplasty. The lateral nasal osteotomies can be performed with an internal or external or even through a transoral approach in some cases. Tip rhinoplasty is best accessed through an external rhinoplasty for the novice, but with time, tip rhinoplasty can be predictable through an internal approach. Nasal base surgery is seldom needed but a valuable tool for the cosmetic surgeon.

REFERENCES

1. Austermann K. Rhinoplasty: planning techniques and complications. In: Booth PW, Hansamen JE, editors. Maxillofacial surgery. New York: Churchill Livingston; 1999. p. 1334–76.
2. Adamson PA, Galli SK. Rhinoplasty approaches: current state of the art. Arch Facial Plast Surg 2005;7:32.
3. Koehler J. Basic rhinoplasty, oral and maxillofacial surgery, vol. 3. St Louis (MO): Elsevier; 2009. p. 553–78.
4. Gunter JP, Landecker A, Cochran CS. Frequently used grafts in rhinoplasty: nomenclature and analysis. Plast Reconstr Surg 2006;118:14e.
5. Staffel JG. Basic principles of rhinoplasty. San Antonio (TX): UTHSCSA; 1996.
6. Ortiz-Monasterio F. Rhinoplasty. Philadelphia: WB Saunder Co; 1994.
7. Kamer FM, Pieper PG. Nasal tip surgery: a 30-year experience. Facial Plast Surg Clin North Am 2004; 12:81.
8. Beeson W, McCollough EG. Aesthetic surgery of the aging face. St Louis (MO): C.V. Mosley Co; 1986.
9. David AM, Simons RL, Rhee JS. Evaluation of the Goldman tip procedure in modern-day rhinoplasty. Arch Facial Plast Surg 2004;6(5): 301–7.
10. Thomas R, Tardy ME. Alar reduction and sculpture, essentials of septorhinoplasty: philosophy approaches, techniques. New York: Thieme; 2004.

Revision Rhinoplasty

Angelo Cuzalina, MD, DDS[a],*, Clement Qaqish, DDS, MD[b]

KEYWORDS

- Revision • Rhinoplasty • Under-resection • Over-resections
- Grafting

Although rhinoplasty is arguably the most challenging of all cosmetic facial procedures, the experience and skill level of a surgeon can significantly affect outcome. Whether novice or seasoned, there are select cases in rhinoplasty that pose significant challenges to the surgeon regardless of experience level. It is through experience and an adequate fund of knowledge that will enable the rhinoplasty surgeon to identify these cases at the time of consultation and plan accordingly. This planning not only involves surgical preparation but also developing a clear understanding of the patient's concerns and educating the patient on what can be realistically achieved.

No cosmetic procedure mandates a thorough preoperative evaluation like rhinoplasty. This is even more imperative in cases of revision rhinoplasty. A complete examination, well documented, including remarks about the patient's esthetic and functional concerns is imperative. A certain subset of patients will never be content with their outcome and will seek revision for small insignificant traits. Most of these patients have body dysmorphic disorder and surgery in these patients should be avoided.[1] Speculum examination is imperative to evaluate the septum for a potential graft source and for irregularities and contour deformities that would warrant correction. Old operative reports, if available, can be useful in surgical planning as well. All patients undergoing primary rhinoplasty should be aware of the risk of the need for revisional surgery. Revision rates reported in the literature are far from insignificant (8%–15%), with experts in the field quoting their own revision rates to be 5% to 10%.[2,3]

TIMING

Patients seeking revision rhinoplasty usually present for consultation 1 year postoperatively. This is in large part because of what is promulgated among rhinoplasty surgeons: soft tissues take approximately 1 year to mature and residual deformities will often resolve. This is not always true, however, and a cohort of patients are satisfied with the surgical result for years before they can appreciate residual deformity. This is largely because of scar contracture or the "shrink wrapping" phenomenon observed in the skin-soft tissue envelope over time.[4] The authors advocate that it is usually wise to wait 1 year before secondary procedures are undertaken. This permits resolution of soft tissue edema and reassessment of deformities should they continue to be a concern. A few exceptions are gross postoperative findings, including saddle nose deformities, airway compromise, and severe loss of tip support, which will likely get worse over the course of a year secondary to scar contracture. Loss of tissue planes will also make delayed revision more difficult. In these instances, earlier operative intervention may yield better results.

We partition this discussion of revisional surgery based on perceived problems with the primary rhinoplasty. This will focus on either underresection or overresection of tissues and the ensuing clinical result. We also discuss some select problems associated with manipulation of tissues via suturing or grafting and briefly discuss functional considerations in secondary surgery. The authors advocate an open approach when performing most revision rhinoplasty. A closed approach may suffice for

[a] 7322 East 91 Street South, Tulsa, OK 74133, USA
[b] Private Practice, North County Cosmetic Surgery, 839 East Grand Avenue, Escondido, CA 92025, USA
* Corresponding author.
E-mail address: angelo@tulsasurgicalarts.com

Oral Maxillofacial Surg Clin N Am 24 (2012) 119–130
doi:10.1016/j.coms.2011.10.003
1042-3699/12/$ – see front matter © 2012 Published by Elsevier Inc.

Normal Nose

Noses with 'Pollybeak Deformities

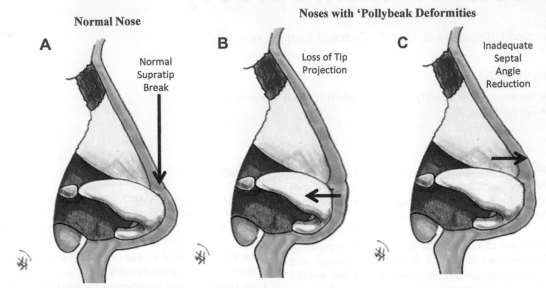

Fig. 1. The pollybeak deformity is one of the most common complications requiring revision. (*A*) A normal nasal profile demonstrates an ideal supratip break. (*B*) A pollybeak deformity that is created by loss of nasal tip projection relative to the area of the anterior septal angle. (*C*) A pollybeak deformity created by inadequate removal of the lower cartilaginous septal portion of a dorsal hump (*Courtesy of* Angelo Cuzalina, MD, DDS, Tulsa, OK.).

correction of certain problems, such as isolated correction of minor irregularities by reduction or grafting. Visualization and access provided by the open approach enables the surgeon to achieve treatment goals in a more predictable fashion, however, particularly in cases requiring extensive grafting or when a different surgeon performed the previous rhinoplasty.

UNDERRESECTION

The notion that it is safer to remove less than more is a surgical mantra ascribed to by many. We examine here the results of underresection of the nasal dorsum, radix, and anterior caudal septum. The most common specific aim in primary rhinoplasty is dorsal hump reduction. The nasal dorsum

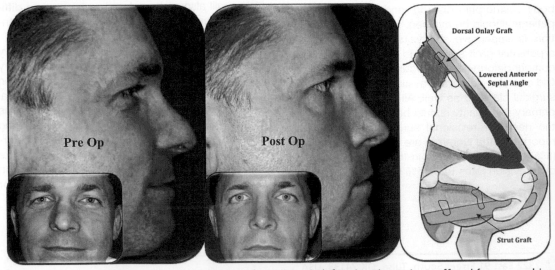

Fig. 2. A 44-year-old before and after treatment of a pollybeak deformity. The patient suffered from a combination of problems, including overresection of the dorsum at the radix, underresection of the cartilaginous septum at the "anterior septal angle," and slight loss of nasal tip support with tip ptosis. Corrective surgery included lowering the septal angle, augmenting the radix region and increasing tip projection by a strut and transdomal sutures (*Courtesy of* Angelo Cuzalina, MD, DDS, Tulsa, OK.).

consists of a bony upper vault and a middle cartilaginous vault. Patients with a prominent nasal dorsum generally have excesses in both areas. Attempts to reduce the hump may involve rasping, osteotomies, and, rarely, grafting.[5]

A pollybeak deformity (**Fig. 1**) is one of the most common reasons for revisional rhinoplasty. Most case series report pollybeak deformity as the primary reason for revision in 40% to 64% of cases.[6–8] The deformity is seen when the area of the supratip break projects ahead of the nasal tip in the plane of the nasal dorsum. This gives the illusion of a bulbous ptotic tip with no supratip break. Two reasons are primarily responsible for this: underresection of the dorsum in the region of the supratip (anterior septal angle) and disruption of the tip supporting structures resulting in depression of the nasal tip postoperatively.[9] Correction of the problem obviates the need to identify the etiology. In cases of underresection at the anterior septal angle, reduction can be easily performed (**Fig. 2**). In cases of disruption of tip-supporting structures, tip support must be obtained by other means. Support may be lost during primary rhinoplasty for several reasons, such as overresected lower lateral cartilages, disarticulation of lower lateral cartilages from the caudal septum, scroll area violation (as in closed approaches), dome division without reapproximation of lower lateral cartilages, disruption of the membranous septum, as seen in hemi or complete transfixion incisions, or simply a lack of additional supporting struts when indicted for poor tissue quality.[10] The loss of tip projection and resultant supratip fullness may lead the novice surgeon to resect more anterior caudal septum when it may instead be necessary to increase tip projection with various grafting techniques.

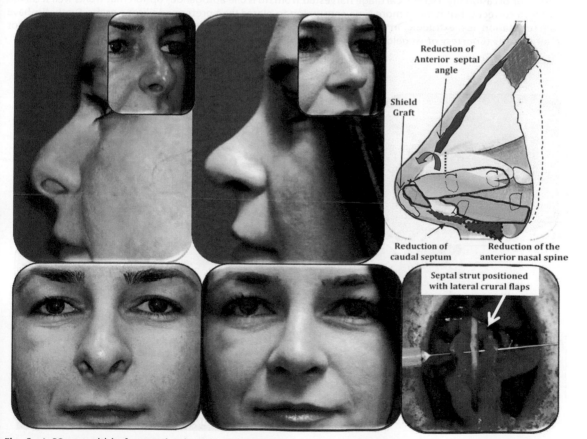

Fig. 3. A 32-year-old before and 1 month after an open rhinoplasty and treatment of a pollybeak deformity secondary to apparent overresection of the tip-supporting elements. The previous surgery also produced severe alar retraction. The result was worsened by underreduction of the anterior septal angle, a hanging columella, and a large anterior nasal spine. A sturdy strut and batten grafts were placed for correction along with rotation of lateral crural flaps (lateral crural steal) to the strut to further increase tip projection. A shield graft further increased tip projection (*Courtesy of* Angelo Cuzalina, MD, DDS, Tulsa, OK.).

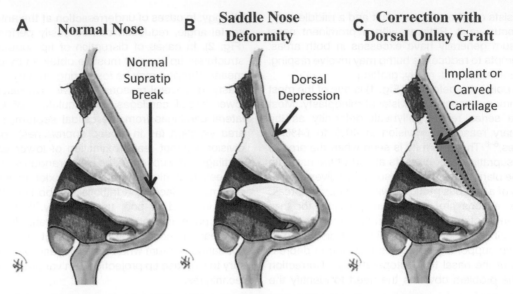

A Normal Nose

Normal Supratip Break

B Saddle Nose Deformity

Dorsal Depression

C Correction with Dorsal Onlay Graft

Implant or Carved Cartilage

Fig. 4. (*A*) Normal nasal dorsal anatomy. (*B*) A "saddle nose" deformity often created by previous surgery or trauma. (*C*) The position of a dorsal onlay graft can be seen in shaded in green. Any graft ideally should be fixed by suture or occasionally a screw. Cartilage harvested from rib is one autogenous option that works well if carved and placed correctly, but is much more time consuming to placed than preformed silicone grafts. Synthetics have a bad reputation for extruding in some surgical circles. Poor-quality tissue is usually a contraindication for synthetic grafts (*Courtesy of* Angelo Cuzalina, MD, DDS, Tulsa, OK.).

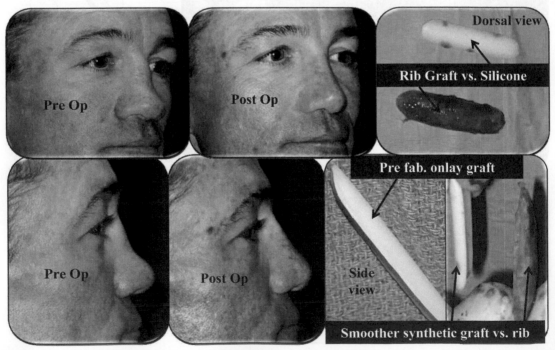

Pre Op

Post Op

Dorsal view

Rib Graft vs. Silicone

Pre fab. onlay graft

Pre Op

Post Op

Side view

Smoother synthetic graft vs. rib

Fig. 5. A 39-year-old with a saddle nose deformity shown preoperatively and 2 years following dorsal onlay grafting using a prefabricated silicon implant. The alternative choice is a meticulously carved cartilage graft (usually from harvest rib) as shown in the figure. Autogenous freeze-dried rib may be used. Measurements should be first taken for the desired length of graft typically placed from nasion to the supratip break. A side-by-side comparison can be used if needed to help better shape a free-hand carved portion of cartilage (*Courtesy of* Angelo Cuzalina, MD, DDS, Tulsa, OK.).

Procedurally, in the context of revision, fashioning of a columellar strut and securing the medial crura of the lower lateral cartilages to the strut will help ameliorate issues with tip support weakening in addition to adding tip projection if desired (**Fig. 3**).

OVERRESECTION

Even with increasing support for preservationalist philosophies and the reliance on tip refinement suturing, the stigmata of overresection in rhinoplasty is still fairly prevalent. The nasal dorsum is often excessively reduced. Perhaps one of the more difficult sequlae resulting from overresection, is a saddle nose deformity or the "scooped out look" (**Fig. 4**). This defect is easily recognizable and its etiology, when septal support is adequate, is almost always related to excessive dorsal reduction. Restoration of form often involves nasal dorsal reconstruction in the form of a dorsal onlay graft (**Fig. 5**).[11] Materials used for dorsal augmentation (and all grafting for that matter) fall into 1 of 3 categories: alloplastic implants, autografts, and allografts. The most commonly used alloplastic implants are silastic, Gore-tex and Medpor grafts. Alloplastic implants are more prone to infection, mobility, and extrusion than autogenous or allogeneic grafts.[12] Allogeneic or homografts (irradiated homograft costal cartilage) are more prone to resorption than alloplasts, with reported resorption rates as high as 11%.[13] Autogenous grafts are the ideal donor site material in terms of immunogenicity with minimal infection rates.[14] The obvious drawback with autograft use is the associated donor site morbidity. In addition, larger grafts have been known to warp over time.[15] Sources for autogenous cartilage include septal, auricular, and costal cartilage. It is prudent in the preoperative clinical examination to determine if septal cartilage was previously harvested as well as having a working knowledge of the stock of cartilage required to achieve treatment goals. Generally, dorsal augmentation requires costal cartilage to be harvested (**Fig. 6**).

Even minimal dorsal hump reduction has the potential to create an open roof deformity (**Fig. 7**), where the nasal bridge appears widened and artificially flat. Topographically, the nasal dorsum is a trapezoid rather than a gently curved triangle. Generally, the dorsal septum can be palpated along with its disjunction from the leading edge of the nasal bone. This is because of

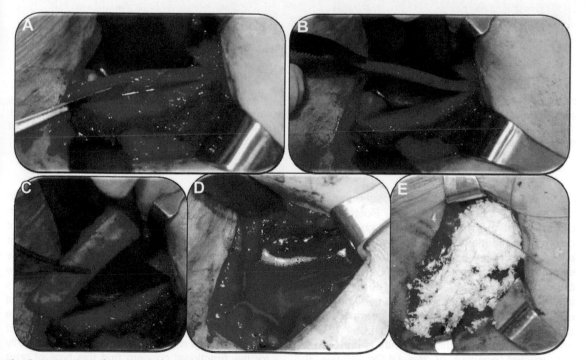

Fig. 6. Harvesting rib cartilage for nasal reconstruction is a common practice when large amounts of sturdy cartilagenous material is required. (*A*) and (*B*) demonstrate protection below the right medial sixth rib with a ribbon retractor to take only the portion of rib desired. (*C*) shows a middle strut of rib often used for tip struts. The outer rounded portion of rib would be left intact for dorsal grafts. After harvest, water in the pocket verifies no bubbles (*D*) and no pneumothorax. Additional hemostasis, accomplished using material such as Avitene, (*E*) helps prevent postoperative hematomas and seromas (*Courtesy of* Angelo Cuzalina, MD, DDS, Tulsa, OK.).

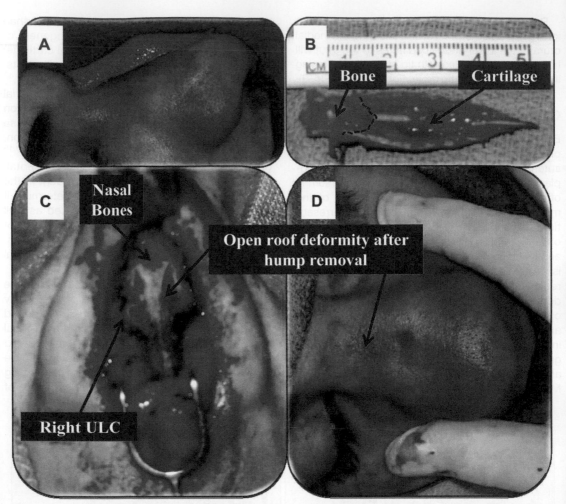

Fig. 7. (*A, B*) The removal of a large dorsal hump of paired nasal bones, paired upper lateral cartilage (ULC), and dorsal septal cartilage. The open rhinoplasty clearly demonstrates the internal "open roof" (*C*) deformity after hump removal. The large open roof is seen externally (*D*) immediately before lateral osteotomies to close and correct the open roof defect, thereby narrowing the upper and middle nasal bridge (*Courtesy of* Angelo Cuzalina, MD, DDS, Tulsa, OK.).

inadequate medialization of the nasal bones when osteotomies are performed.[10,11] Postosteotomy palpation of the redraped skin to check for any dorsal irregularities will ameliorate this problem in either the primary or secondary rhinoplasty. Inadequate medialization of the nasal bones may also cause an inverted V deformity (**Fig. 8**), where a sharp delineation is seen between the caudal end of the nasal bones and the cephalic margin of the upper lateral cartilages (ULCs).[16,17] The anatomic reason for this deformity is consistently the medial position of the ULCs relative the nasal bones. In cases of excessive middle vault resection, the tendency is for the ULCs to destabilize and collapse medially. This medial positioning is exacerbated by the thinner septum that remains after trimming.[4] Prevention is centered

on completion of adequate osteotomies or middle vault reconstruction with proper resuspension of the ULCs to the dorsal septum. In cases of excessive middle vault resection, the placement of spreader grafts may be necessary to recreate the natural flare seen in the topography of the middle vault (**Fig. 9**). Spreader cartilaginous grafts placed between the septum and upper lateral cartilages may be used as a preventive measure in patients with high narrow vaults who are at risk for internal nasal valve collapse. It is primarily for this functional concern that this type of graft is placed.[18,19]

Cephalic strips are often taken in an attempt to refine a nasal tip lobule. Excessive removal with associated weakening of the bridging lower lateral crus (LLC), and dead space, creates a

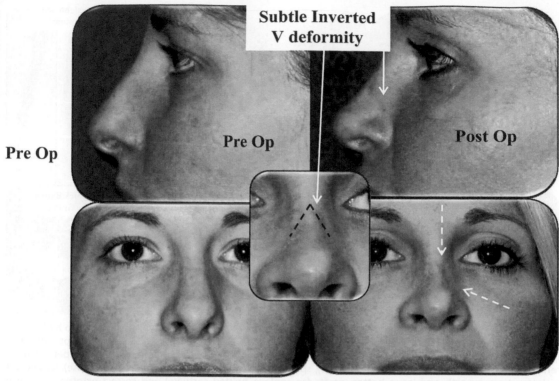

Fig. 8. A 35-year-old woman before and 5 years following rhinoplasty and orthognathic surgery. Her thin nasal skin demonstrates a subtle "inverted V" deformity seen as a light shadow depression along the connection between ULC and the nasal bones. Treatment can range from no treatment to injectable fillers or revisional lateral osteotomies and lateralizing ULC in severe cases (*Courtesy of* Angelo Cuzalina, MD, DDS, Tulsa, OK.).

situation where scar contracture can pull up on the cartilaginous arch resulting in alar retraction (**Fig. 10**).[16] Overresection of tissues, as a cause of retraction, needs to be discerned from previously placed rim or caudally placed marginal incisions for surgical access. Management of alar retraction (the classic "piggy" or "gun barrel" nose), involves bolstering the lower lateral cartilages with batten grafts, as is done for external valve collapse (**Fig. 11**).[20] External valve collapse

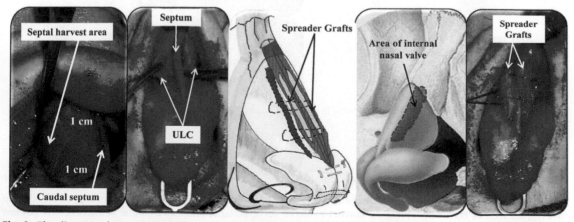

Fig. 9. The diagrams demonstrate each aspect of placement of cartilagenous septal grafts and spreader grafts beginning with harvesting septal cartilage and leaving adequate superior and anterior support. The spreader grafts are placed in a pocket created between the ULC and the dorsal septum (*Courtesy of* Angelo Cuzalina, MD, DDS, Tulsa, OK.).

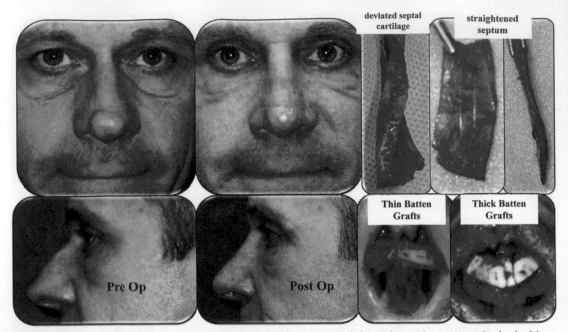

Fig. 10. A 52-year-old man shown before and 6 weeks after revisional rhinoplasty. The patient also had a history a nasal trauma and reports severe bilateral breathing compromise. His examination revealed septal deviation, and external nasal valve and severe internal nasal valve collapse along with a twisted nose. The patient underwent total nasal reconstruction with septoplasty, spreader grafts (to correct external valve collapse), large caudal strut (for tip support), and large batten grafts (to replace twisted cartilage and correct external nasal valve collapse) (*Courtesy of* Angelo Cuzalina, MD, DDS, Tulsa, OK.).

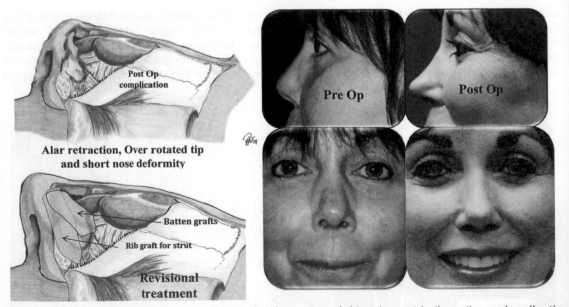

Fig. 11. A 63-year-old woman before and 8 months after revisional rhinoplasty with rib cartilage columellar-tip grafting, as well as batten grafting, to correct external valve collapse and extreme alar retraction. The patient reported having 2 previous septorhinoplasties years prior. Rib cartilage was selected for strength, size, and lack of other suitable cartilage required in tertiary noses. The patient also had a severe "inverted-V" deformity that required corrective complete lateral osteotomies (*Courtesy of* Angelo Cuzalina, MD, DDS, Tulsa, OK.).

is a commonly missed diagnosis. Reinforcing of the lateral crus provides support for the weakened and collapsible sidewall observed in this deformity.

SHORT NOSE

The overshortened nose is one of the most difficult sequelae to repair. It is often the result of excessive resection of the caudal septum, resulting in overrotation of the nasal tip as healing and scar contractures evolve. Repair often involves placement of caudal septal extension grafts, extension spreader grafts, and often columellar and alar grafting (**Fig. 12**).[21]

TIP REVISION

The nasal tip presents unique problems in both primary and secondary rhinoplasty. The tip is the most variable anatomic part of the nose. The lower lateral cartilages are often asymmetric with overlying soft tissues of varying thickness. There are a multitude of tip-related indications for revision rhinoplasty. Among these is a pinched nasal tip, the appearance of which is self-explanatory (**Fig. 13**). This problem is caused by

either overapproximation of the domes at the conclusion of the primary procedure and/or soft tissue contracture overlying an insufficient tip framework classically caused by overresection of LLCs. Correction, best achieved with an open approach, should be centered on grafting. Shield grafts can provide adequate bulk to the tip; however, caution must be exercised in patients with thin skin who, over time, are more prone to development of bossae (contour irregularities in the tip).[22,23] One way to treat or prevent bossae formation is to carefully contour and soften all grafts placed. In addition, coverage with a dermal allograft may be helpful in preventing these irregularities from developing.[24]

FUNCTIONAL ISSUES

In revision rhinoplasty, the stability of the nasal valves is often in question. Surgery of the middle vault will often compromise the internal nasal valve. Medialization of the cartilages as a result of reductive procedures and removal of the dorsal septal flare contribute to restriction of flows through the valve.[25] This is exacerbated by scar contraction. Performing a Cottle test preoperatively will confirm

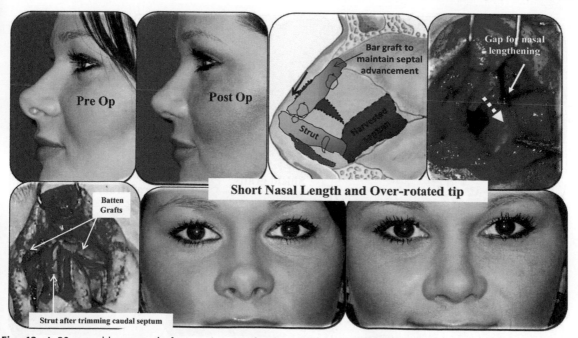

Fig. 12. A 20-year-old woman before and 1 month after an open septorhinoplasty to correct a short nose as measured from radix to nasal tip. The nose was lengthened by separating the anterior septum and advancing it caudally using a "septal bar" graft to span the defect and maintain caudal displacement of the dorsal septum. Batten onlay grafts were used to help lengthen the nose at the alar rim and decrease nostril show. A large caudal strut graft was sutured to the caudal septum securely and tip forward to de-rotate the nasal tip. Excess caudal septum below the tip was trimmed to further treat the hanging columella (*Courtesy of* Angelo Cuzalina, MD, DDS, Tulsa, OK.).

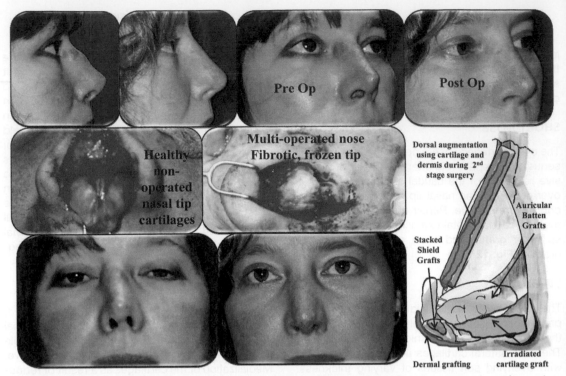

Fig. 13. A 38-year-old woman before and 4 years after staged open rhinoplasty reconstruction. The patient reportedly had more than 10 previous nasal surgeries and presented with an infected Gore-tex dorsal graft. The initial surgery consisted of exploration and debridement of infected graft with limited nasal vestibular skin grafts and dermal augmentation. Second-stage surgery 3 months later involved major grafting using auricular cartilage for batten grafts and dorsal augmentation along with irradiated rib cartilage grafting and dermal grafting. No significant septal cartilage was present and she preferred irradiated cartilage over a rib harvest (*Courtesy of* Angelo Cuzalina, MD, DDS, Tulsa, OK.).

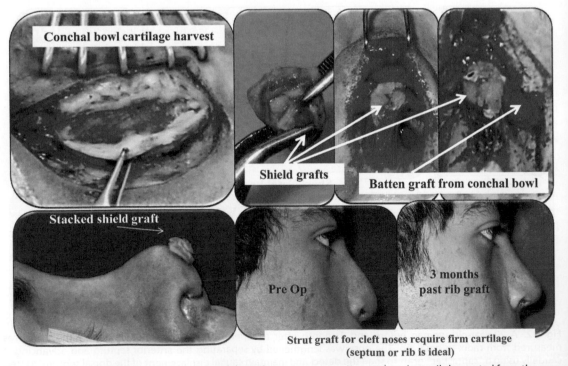

Fig. 14. Auricular cartilage has a better natural shape for alar reconstruction and can be easily harvested from the cymba concha via a postauricular crease incision as shown. This useful cartilage is great for shield and batten grafts, as demonstrated in this figure. Noses scarred previously, however, like the patient with cleft lip and palate in this figure, require much stronger cartilage, such as rib or septum to significantly increase projection (*Courtesy of* Angelo Cuzalina, MD, DDS, Tulsa, OK.).

the need for reconstitution of the internal valve dimension. Placement of spreader grafts prophylactically, or at the time of revision, will either prevent or ameliorate this problem.

Cephalic strips are often taken to help sculpt the nasal tip. Excessive removal of the lower lateral cartilages not only results in unsightly notching and alar retraction, as previously noted, but this is often the cause of external valve collapse. Correction of this deformity almost always involves grafting. Auricular cartilage has a better natural shape for alar reconstruction.[26] These grafts can be easily harvested from the cymba concha via an anterior or posterior approach (**Fig. 14**). They may be placed as alar battens on top of existing cartilage, or as struts between the cartilage and the mucosa. If the alar rim contour is questionable, an alar rim graft may also be used to restore natural alar curvature.

SCARRING

Although the open approach has made the correction of many nasal deformities more predictable, the potential for scarring of the columellar incision is ever present. The proper placement of the incision, either inverted-V or stair step, gentle tissue handling, and meticulous closure are all critical to minimize scarring. Scar revision in this area is difficult and may yield even more unfavorable results. The scarring associated with alar base resection and the alar notching associated with a rim incision or poorly placed marginal incisions, are also a surgical dilemma. Proper incision placement is the rule, and alar base incisions should not be made in natural creases and should never extend beyond the natural alar curve. We advocate a more internal placement of these incisions, within the confines of the nasal sill.

SUMMARY

As the number of surgeons performing rhinoplasty grows, the experience level of the average surgeon potentially decreases. It is not surprising then that the revision rate of rhinoplasty is as high as it is. This problem is exacerbated by unrealistic patient expectations, largely cultivated by the media, and at times the optimistic assertions of the surgeons themselves. Frankly, the procedure itself is technically more difficult than most procedures. Revision rhinoplasty encompasses a wide range of clinical presentations. There are a multitude of potential problems requiring correction. The surgeon is not only dealing with these physical factors but also the psyche of the patient, whose confidence in the surgeon may be less than ideal. When it comes to revision rhinoplasty, it is far better to under promise and over deliver. One cannot divorce form and function. An astute awareness of functional compromise and its correction is as important as achieving esthetic goals. Experience with several techniques and approaches will aid the surgeon in better serving this challenging patient cohort.

REFERENCES

1. Sarwer DB, Crerand CE, Didie ER. Body dysmorphic disorder in cosmetic surgery patients. Facial Plast Surg 2003;19:7–18.
2. Mazzola RF, Felisati G. Secondary rhinoplasty: analysis of the deformity and guidelines for management. Facial Plast Surg 1997;13:163–77.
3. Quatela VC, Jacono AA. Structural grafting in rhinoplasty. Facial Plast Surg 2002;18:223–32.
4. Tardy ME. Rhinoplasty: the art and the science. Philadelphia: WB Saunders; 1997.
5. Steigler JD, Baker SR. Nuances of profile management: the radix. Facial Plast Surg Clin North Am 2009;17:15–28.
6. Foda HM. Rhinoplasty for the multiply revised nose. Am J Otolaryngol 2005;26:28–34.
7. Vuyk HD, Watts SJ, Vindayak B. Revision rhinoplasty: review of deformities, aetiology, and treatment strategies. Clin Otolaryngol Allied Sci 2000;25:476–81.
8. Kamer FM, McQuown SA. Revision rhinoplasty. Analysis and treatment. Arch Otolaryngol Head Neck Surg 1988;114:257–66.
9. Cuzalina A. Rhinoplasty. In: Niamtu J, editor. Cosmetic facial surgery. St Louis (MO): Mosby Elsevier; 2011. p. 175–246.
10. Chrostophel JJ, Park SS. Complications in rhinoplasty. Facial Plast Surg Clin North Am 2009;17:145–56.
11. Papel ID. Facial plastic and reconstructive surgery. 3rd edition. New York: Thieme; 2009.
12. Adamson PA. Grafts in rhinoplasty: autogenous grafts are superior to alloplastic. Arch Otolaryngol Head Neck Surg 2000;126(4):561–2.
13. Burke AJ, Wang TD, Cook TA. Irradiated homograft rib cartilage in facial reconstruction. Arch Facial Plast Surg 2004;6:334–41.
14. Kridel RW, Kraus WM. Grafts and implants in revision rhinoplasty. Facial Plast Surg Clin North Am 1995;3:473–86.
15. Kim DW, Shah AR, Toriumu DM. Concentric and eccentric carved costal cartilage: a comparison of warping. Arch Facial Plast Surg 2006;8:42–6.
16. Toriumi DM. Rhinoplasty. In: Park SS, editor. Facial plastic surgery: the essential guide. New York: Thieme; 2005. p. 80–96.
17. Rohrich RJ, Muzaffar AR, Janis JE. Component dorsal hump reduction: the importance of maintaining

dorsal aesthetic lines in rhinoplasty. Plast Reconstr Surg 2004;114:1298–308.

18. Park SS, Becker SS. Repair of nasal airway obstruction in revision rhinoplasty. In: Becker DG, Park SS, editors. Revision rhinoplasty. New York: Thieme; 2008. p. 60–76.

19. Sheen J. Spreader graft: a method of reconstructing the middle nasal vault following rhinoplasty. Plast Reconstr Surg 1984;73(2):230–9.

20. Toriumi DM, Josen J, Weinberger M, et al. Use of alar batten grafts for correction of nasal valve collapse. Arch Otolaryngol Head Neck Surg 1997; 123(8):802–8.

21. Gruber RP. Surgical correction of the short nose. Aesthetic Plast Surg 2002;26(Suppl 1):6.

22. Adamson PA, Little JA. Revision tip rhinoplasty. In: Becker DG, Park SS, editors. Revision rhinoplasty. New York: Thieme; 2008. p. 77–89.

23. Gilman GS, Simons RL, Lee DJ. Nasal tip bossae in rhinoplasty: etiology, predisposing factors and management techniques. Arch Facial Plast Surg 1999;1:83–9.

24. Gryskiewicz JM, Rohrich RJ, Reagan BJ. The use of alloderm for the correction of nasal contour deformities. Plast Reconstr Surg 2001;107:561–70.

25. Fischer H, Gubisch W. Nasal valves—importance and surgical procedures. Facial Plast Surg 2006;22: 49–54.

26. Murrell GL. Auricular cartilage grafts and nasal surgery. Laryngoscope 2004;114:2092–102.

Ethnic Rhinoplasty

Mohan Thomas, MD, DDS[a,b],*, James D'Silva, MCH, DNB[a,b]

KEYWORDS

- Rhinoplasty • Ethnic patients • Surgical planning
- Complications

Ethnology may be a fascinating subject; however, it remains academic for the most part. The classification of noses into leptorrhines (narrow), platyrrhines (broad), and mesorrhines (somewhere in between) along with the calculation of the nasal index or comparison of cephalometric findings may be interesting if one is engaged in anthropometric studies.[1]

When considering rhinoplasty in ethnic patients one must determine their aesthetic goals, which in many cases might deviate from the so-called norm of the "North European nose."

Although the earliest recorded facial proportion analysis is found in the Greek neoclassical canons (ca 450 BC), in modern times there has been no study that adequately describes the relative differences in facial proportions among the world's different ethnic groups.[2] The neoclassical canons included heights and widths of the upper, middle, and lower face. A review of the literature shows the greatest interethnic variability in facial proportions to exist in the height of the forehead. In the ethnic groups the most pronounced differences are present in the dimensions of the eyes, nose, and mouth, whereas no significant differences were present between the sexes in the neoclassical facial proportions.[3]

The term ethnic rhinoplasty has been used rather loosely to describe any nose other than the Caucasian nose, such as the African American nose, Hispanic nose, Asian nose, Middle Eastern nose, Indian nose, and others from the same subcontinent. It is perhaps more important to understand what the different characteristics of the various ethnicities are, rather than to develop an algorithm for the management of the various problems of patients at presentation. Statistics indicate that more than 3 million cosmetic plastic surgery procedures were performed on ethnic patients in 2009, with an increase of approximately about 215% since 2000. Facial plastic surgeons have seen the largest increase in the number of African American, Asian, and Hispanic patients in 2010.[4]

There is a paucity in ethnic diversity in academic plastic, reconstructive, and cosmetic surgery. Among the United States residents/fellows, 68.7% are Caucasians while Asian, African, and Latin Americans comprise 20.9%, 3.7%, and 6.2%, respectively. In the academic scenario Caucasians comprise 74.9% while the Asian, African, and Latin Americans constitute 10.9%, 1.4%, and 3.6%, respectively. It is clear that a larger number of ethnic surgeons as well as surgeons familiar with ethnicity are required to establish a health care environment that is more accommodating for the minority patients as well as to provide role models and mentors.[5,6]

According to Jack H. Sheen, "there is logic in the selection since the various ethnicities share many common anatomic similarities." Norman Rappaport states that substantial tip grafts, alar excisions, and remodeling of the rest of the nose for balance form the basis for a surgical correction of the ethnic nasal deformity, as perceived by the patient. He further stresses that the rate of revision for ethnic noses may be double that for Caucasian noses. Alarming as it may seem, the take-home message is the need for appropriate evaluation of a patient and preoperative counseling, particularly with regard to his or her expectations.[7]

AESTHETIC CONSIDERATIONS IN ETHNIC RHINOPLASTY

The elements of beauty are universal and generally involve harmony, balance, regularity, and poise.

[a] The Cosmetic Surgery Institute, 169, Lily Villa, St Andrews Road, Bandra-West, Mumbai, Maharashtra, India 400050

[b] Cosmetic Surgery, Breach Candy Hospital, Mumbai, Maharashtra, India

* Corresponding author. The Cosmetic Surgery Institute, 169, Lily Villa, St Andrews Road, Bandra-West, Mumbai, Maharashtra, India 400050.

E-mail address: drmohan.thomas@gmail.com

Oral Maxillofacial Surg Clin N Am 24 (2012) 131–148

doi:10.1016/j.coms.2011.11.003

1042-3699/12/$ – see front matter © 2012 Elsevier Inc. All rights reserved.

The tenets of rhinoplasty that provide a basis for any surgical plan remain the same regardless of the ethnic origin of the patients. The nose, being the center stage of the face, can appear larger, wider, thicker, longer, or higher than what is considered an accepted norm, and must be in harmony with the face or type of face, so that it is considered attractive in a theoretical sense. Beauty is in the eyes of the beholder and therefore assessment, surgical procedures, and outcomes must be practical. The so-called standards of beauty that have been imprinted on our society by the mass media and film personalities are generally of the northern European type. These noses have been portrayed as being straight with a narrow nasal bridge, a well-defined and projecting nasal tip, alar refinement, and a nasolabial angle of about 90°. Those who belong to the ethnic minorities may feel set apart under the pressure of these standards, and some of them may even feel at a disadvantage because of their "nonstandard appearance." Others may feel differently in a positive way and identify themselves with a particular group. These patients may desire nasal alterations to bring them closer to what they have come to accept as beautiful or desirable. At this point one must exert great caution. The cosmetic objective of the person who desires to blend in, and look like the majority, are radically different from the person who wishes to have a more attractive nose without losing ethnic character. These desires and expectations need to be clearly understood preoperatively so that the operation will be appropriate.

There are two common issues that one must deal. In the first scenario a patient's rhinoplastic change may make him or her lose his or her ethnicity, resulting in loss of identity. In the second scenario the patient wants a change or elimination of ethnic features, which may be impossible because of anatomic and tissue limitations. These cases need to be well recognized and carefully managed to avoid serious disappointment and dissatisfaction of the patient.

THE ETHNIC GROUPS

In an article on ethnic rhinoplasty it is important that the different ethnic groups are delineated. The word ethnic has often been used to lump together all subsets other than Caucasian. The authors redefine these types as the African American, the Latin American, the Middle Eastern, the Asian, and variations of the Middle Eastern nose from countries in South Asia. In this article the authors attempt to pinpoint the most common shared features of each of these groups to help in the surgical planning, keeping in mind the nuances of the various ethnic groups.

It is not within the scope of this article either to describe all of the variations and subsets of the ethnic groups or to provide a surgical algorithm. The information herein will help the clinician to narrow down the surgical choices depending on the ethnicity, adding one's own aesthetic angle and not forgetting the patient's personal desires. It is important that the patient has a realistic expectations, and he or she must understand changes that are not possible even more clearly than what is possible.

In addition, one has to deal with the very strong anatomic structures and individual skin cover, which is often thick and sebaceous, not to mention concerns about hyperpigmentation and scarring, as most of these ethnic groups except the Asians are rated 4, 5, or 6 on the Fitzpatrick scale.

The Fibrofatty Layer

The fibrofatty tissue plays a dominant role in the appearance of some of the ethnic groups mentioned such as the African American, some Latin American, and most Middle Eastern and South Asian noses. The preponderance of this fatty layer, usually found overlying the lower lateral cartilages and in between the medial crura, is responsible for the poor definition and floppiness of the tip. Care should be taken when skeletonizing the lower lateral cartilages that aggressive removal from the overlying skin does not injure the dermal plexus, which may lead to necrosis or hyperpigmented areas.

Elimination of any or all dead space after any refinement or definition of the nasal tip is critical because recurrences of the same bulky or droopy tip can occur, due to a tendency for excessive scarring. It is also essential that one maintains meticulous hemostasis, as any pooling of blood will result in excessive scarring as well (**Fig. 1**).

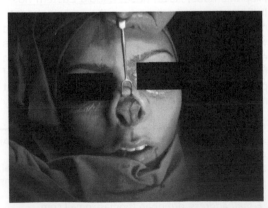

Fig. 1. The prominent fibrofatty layer over the lower lateral cartilages, plunging in between the medial crura.

The African American Nose

There appears to be a great deal of variation in this ethnic group, mainly due to the Arab and Atlantic slave trades beginning in the ninth and fifteenth centuries.[8] Undoubtedly this represents one of the largest migrations in human history and is most likely responsible for the confluence of multiple races and ethnicities throughout the world. African traits seem to have exerted influence worldwide, leading to similarities among African Americans, Hispanics, Arabs, and people from the West Indies.

Most common anatomic presentation

The typical African American nose is flattened and has an increased alar width. The pyriform aperture is wide and forms the skeletal basis for the wide base of the nose. A lack of profile of the nasal dorsum does exist, as there is some degree of natural saddling of the dorsum.[9,10] The tip is flat and round with a significant lack of projection, obviously due to a decrease in the length of the columella. In addition to the ala being flared, the nostrils are large and rounded; there is often an acute columellar-labial angle due to some retraction of the columella. Interestingly enough, although scar hypertrophy or true keloid formation is quite common in this group, it is virtually nonexistent even with a transcolumellar inverted "V" incision. Whereas the projection of the septal angle that provides most of the tip projection is often lowered in the Caucasian nose, it generally needs to be increased in African American noses. It is also obvious that shortening of the nose or any resection of the inferior margin of the septum is not required during rhinoplasty.

Surgical direction

Open or external rhinoplasty is an excellent choice of surgical approach in such patients for surgeons with expertise in this technique. Ofodile and Bokhari[11,12] advocated the use of open rhinoplasty as well. It is frequently necessary to use a columellar strut graft, often harvested from the nasal septum. In addition, cartilage grafting using the Gunter, Sheen, or Peck technique[13] should be used to improve the nasal tip and give it projection.

Leading rhinoplasty surgeons who are experienced largely or almost exclusively with Caucasians have not endorsed the use of alloplastic materials. It is the opinion of Thomas D. Rees and the senior author (M.T.) that there is a real place for alloplastic augmentation of the dorsum in these and other non-Caucasian noses. A review of more than 250 implants in the authors' practice confirms the long-term acceptability of silicone implants to the nasal dorsum while taking care to leave some soft tissue/periosteum between the implant and the nasal bone. Obviously, whenever possible autogenous tissue is always preferred; however, at times the amount of augmentation necessary often far exceeds the amount of autogenous cartilage available, while bone grafts remain unacceptable to many patients and also have a potential for some amount of resorption.

This group of patients often requires the alar region to be addressed for an increased width of the alar base as well as the alar flare. Surgeries involving alar base reduction are done by performing a nasal sill reduction into the vestibule. The nasal flare reduction needs removal of a wedge of tissue from the alae, and should leave behind 1 to 2 mm of tissue above the alar groove to preserve the vascularity, and also to allow better suturing and a good scar. In the authors' experience greater stability in the management of the alar reduction can be achieved by the use of cinching sutures engaging the soft tissues at the level of the alar base and the foot plates of the lower lateral cartilages.

Skeletally speaking, this group often presents with bimaxillary protrusion and in some cases relative hypoplasia of the mentum. The increased width of the piriform base is discussed elsewhere.

The Asian Nose

Globalization and migration patterns have made the Asian community a significant minority all over the globe, particularly in the United States and many parts of the European Union. As the population increases it becomes important in a multiracial situation that surgeons become familiar with management of the Asian nose.

Most common anatomic presentation

The nasal characteristics that are common are often low dorsa and weak lower lateral cartilages, with usually a thick sebaceous skin cover. There is a tendency for widening of the piriform rim, which in turn results in a relatively wide alar base and presents with a short columella that is inherent in this group. This nose also presents some unique problems such as short nasal bones, which are not conducive to any kind of aggressive osteotomies, lateral or medial. Patients' needs and expectations are quite unique to this group, as they prefer refinement of their Asian features as opposed to more characteristic white features.[14]

Surgical direction

As one of the most common presenting complaints is the depressed dorsum, the use of alloplastic or autologous material is necessary to achieve the desired results. Obviously the benefits and risks involved in the use of such material need to be discussed with the patient. Autologous tissue, such as stacking of septal cartilage encased in Alloderm (LifeCell Corp, Branchburg, NJ, USA) or costal cartilage, can produce excellent long-term results. The volume of augmentation required very often exceeds what is available autologously from the septum, and some patients may be resistant to costal cartilage harvesting even though it is a reliable and low-risk technique. As a result alloplastic materials, particularly prefabricated silicone implants, can be considered. In most Asian patients it is preferable not to perform lateral osteotomies, not only due to anatomic reasons but also to avoid an unnatural vertical transition from the nasal dorsum and side walls to the maxilla.

The lower lateral cartilages are generally poorly defined, weak, and often overlaid with some amount of fibrofatty tissue that further weakens it. A columellar strut graft, harvested preferably from the septum or conchal cartilage, is used to address the retracted columella to which the medial crus of the lower lateral cartilages is sutured to support the tip. Interdomal and/or transdomal sutures may be necessary to further strengthen the nasal tip. Further refinement of the tip, if necessary, can be achieved by additional tip-defining cartilage grafts using the Gunter, Sheen, or Peck technique,[13] or use of a shield graft if the lower lateral cartilages are unusually weak.

In addition, adjunctive procedures to narrow the nasal base and correction of the columellar and premaxillary retraction may be required. The short nose profile and the lack of projection may further be aggravated by hypoplasia of piriform rim base and the premaxillary region, needing augmentation with alloplastic material such as polytetrafluoroethylene (PTFE) or a bone graft, preferably cranial, secured by a screw.

Often the facial skeleton presents with a relative widening of the pyriform rim, ethnically acceptable hypoplasia of the mid face, and a retruded chin.

The Hispanic Nose

There is significant variability in the anatomic characteristics of Hispanic patients, due to the variable heritage of these patients around the world as is true with the African American and Middle Eastern noses. The Hispanic nose has been discussed by Ortiz-Monasterio and Olmeda[15,16] relative to the Mestizo nose and the Chata nose by Sanchez.[17] There also exists an anthropometric analysis of female Latinas by Milgram and colleagues.[18] According to Daniel,[19] irrespective of national origin

3 common nasal deformities exist, with the fourth one being similar to the African American nose.

The diversity within the Hispanic population has led to variable anatomic and morphologic features somewhere between an African American and European nose. Variability exists in skin thickness, tip projection, nasal dorsum, and alar flaring, and frequently there is a broader nasal base.[18–20]

Surgical direction

The extreme variability in this group requires a variety of surgical techniques, which may be augmentative in nature or reductive at times, with correction of overprojected and underprojected tips, creation of a supratip break, and management of the width of the alar base. Occasionally patients may present with a dorsal hump, which the authors prefer to downsize by rasping followed by checking with the skin cover in place. The authors do not recommend the use of osteotomes for removal of the dorsal hump unless the rhinoplastic surgeon is very experienced. Iatrogenic defects can be caused by overresection with an osteotome.

Skeletally speaking, because of the wide variations in presentation the deformities can range from a short face to a long face, skeletal class 2 or 3, or a retrusive or protrusive chin. Appropriate additional surgical measures may be required to bring greater harmony of the face.

The Middle Eastern, Indian, and Other South Asian Noses

People from the Middle Eastern region and Asian Indian subcontinent have now spread all over the world, and there is an increase in the need for rhinoplastic surgeons to understand the physical and social characteristics of this ethnic group. It is important that there is balance between the surgical goal and the ethnic facial features, as otherwise there would be racial incongruity. For the purposes of this discussion Middle Eastern patients refers to people from the North African countries, Gulf countries, and the Indian peninsula. These patients usually want to retain their specific ethnic traits, such as the higher dorsum and less obtuse nasolabial and columellar-labial angles. Most patients are female and like to have a detailed discussion about the surgical plan.[21]

Most common anatomic presentation

The most characteristic presentation of these patients is the presence of a prominent bulbous tip with thick sebaceous skin, especially on the tip. The nasal bones are usually broad with a very prominent hump, which is usually cartilaginous and bony. This hump is also associated with a typical droopy nose, which droops further on smiling because of the prominent effect of the depressor septi nasi muscle. In turn this gives an overprojected look to the nasal tip and also makes the dorsum look more prominent than usual. Sometimes one finds a deficiency of the alar cartilages, causing a weakness in the tip area as well.

Features that are generally less frequent in this group of patients are a low dorsum, inadequate nasal length, thin skin envelope, round or transverse oriented nostrils, and excess nostril show on frontal view.

Surgical direction

This group of patients presents with a wide range of problems, therefore the treatment plans can include reduction of the dorsum and lateral/medial osteotomies to narrow the bony vault.

Defining the nasal tip is often required, which should commence with definition of the lower lateral cartilages by debulking the fibrofatty tissue overlying the cartilages as well as between the medial crura. Interdomal and transdomal suturing of the lower lateral cartilages and a cephalic trim of the lower lateral cartilages is often required. Toriami[22] also places importance on the position of the cephalic lateral crural margin relative to the caudal margin.[23] When the cephalic margin is oriented on a different plane to the caudal margin, inherent lateral crural instability exists, which should always be addressed before tip shaping.[22,24,25] Tip stability is crucial, as postoperative polybeak deformity is not uncommon in this ethnic group. A Gunter type, Sheen type, and/or Peck onlay graft may be indicated.

This is probably the largest group of patients that requires some form of grafting such as columellar strut grafting, baton grafts, or spreader grafts (following aggressive dorsal hump removal resulting in an open-roof deformity). Baton grafts can be used in a caudal position to the lower lateral cartilages to reduce the convexity if it exists, and can also be used to address management of the collapse of the internal valves (a functional improvement) to name but two applications.

One of the greatest challenges in this group of patients is the skin and soft-tissue envelope, which is poorly contractile, thick, and sebaceous. Patients frequently have Fitzpatrick skin types 3 to 6. The skin characteristics of this group are most challenging at the supratip and infratip lobule. The dorsum and nasal tip often exhibit a high degree of sebaceousness. Dermatologic management of the skin using retinoic acid topically and/or orally may be required in severe cases to reduce the density of the sebaceous skin.

Alar flaring and increased interalar width are common. Conservative alar base surgery is highly recommended (if the rim is >2 mm outside the medial canthal line) when the nostrils are normal. The flaring is corrected by limiting the excision to only alar flare. There often exist asymmetries with the alar and nostril position. In alar flaring with excessive nostril size (increased interalar width), a complete wedge excision should be performed extending into the vestibule 2 mm above the alar groove. The hanging columella deformity occurs in this group, due to alar-columellar disharmony,[23] while primary alar retraction or excess nostril show is rare.[26,27] Medial crural septal sutures and caudal septal resection may be required to improve and maintain tip rotation. There is significant concern about tip overrotation, which in this group is probably the most important imbalance to be avoided.

Residual nostril abnormalities become even more apparent if the medial crural foot plates are flared. A short nostril deformity,[28] soft triangle excess or enlarged/improperly angled nostril apertures, is corrected by appropriate suturing. The soft triangle excision and/or tip suturing techniques to elevate the nostril and elongate the nostrils have been well described by Guyuron and colleagues.[28]

The depressor septi nasi muscle is often hypertrophied resulting in a hyperdynamic nasal tip, which is surgically addressed by transection/transposition of the muscle.[29] In an open rhinoplasty procedure this muscle is transected, which may have to be addressed separately under closed rhinoplasty if needed.

Skeletally the presentation is as varied as the group itself, resulting in usually a long face, occasionally a short face, bimaxillary protrusion, skeletal class 2 and 3, and either a solitary retrusive or protrusive chin.

CASE REPORTS
The African American Nose

The overall similarities in the noses of this ethnic group are stark. Frequently their noses are described as platyrhine.[30] In general the African American nose has a wide, depressed dorsum, inadequate tip projection, poorly defined tip, excess alar flare, and/or increased interalar width, thus overall having a reduced nasal length and height.[30,31] The following patients demonstrate most of these characteristics.

Patient 1

This 34-year-old healthy woman presented with the complaint that her nose looked depressed and very wide. She was also concerned about the bulbous shape of the nasal tip.

Preoperative evaluation On frontal view the bony vault appeared broad because of inadequate dorsal height, and a poorly defined and bulbous tip were apparent. The lateral view showed a very low dorsum and a bulbous overprojected tip while the basal view showed the nostrils to be small and oval.

The operative goal was to raise the dorsum, sharpen the tip, change the columellar lip angle, and narrow the dorsum.

Surgical plan

1. Open rhinoplasty
2. Defatting the nasal tip skin for tip definition
3. Augmenting the dorsum using a silastic implant
4. Lateral osteotomy and infracture of the nasal bones for a narrower dorsum
5. Alar base reduction.

In comparison with preoperative views, 1-year postoperative views show a more narrowed and refined nose, with prominent tip projection and a refined tip. The racial characteristics have been maintained (**Fig. 2**).

Patient 2

A 32-year-old woman presented for improvement of the nose with a blunt tip on a flat, poorly defined nose. She also was concerned about the supratip demarcation line, which was hyperpigmented.

Preoperative evaluation On frontal view there was a wide dorsum and alar bases, with a bulbous tip and a very prominent hype pigmented horizontal line in the supratip area. The lateral view showed a depressed dorsum, prominent rounded tip, and an overhanging columellar. The basal view showed a wide alar base and transversally oval alar openings.

The operative goal was to raise the dorsum and improve the tip definition, with reduction in the alar base.

Surgical plan

1. Open rhinoplasty with a transcolumellar incision
2. Defatting the tip to make it less bulbous
3. Cephalic trim of lower lateral cartilage
4. Dorsal augmentation using a silastic implant
5. Alar base reduction.

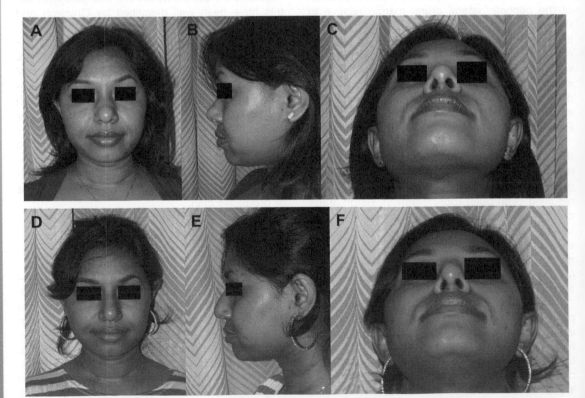

Fig. 2. (A–C) Different preoperative views. (D–F) The same patient 1 year postoperatively.

Preoperative and 3-month postoperative views are shown in **Fig. 3**.

The Asian Nose

Platyrrhine nasal characteristics are common with Asian patients with low dorsum, and weak lower lateral cartilages and thick sebaceous skin are often noted.[13] Patients often seek improvements and refinements of their Asian features without having any radical change to Caucasian looks. Use of alloplasts or autologous materials is needed to achieve the desired results. The following two patients demonstrate these characteristics, and a short treatment plan is provided.

Patient 3

This 42-year-old healthy married patient presented with the complaint that her nose looked too oriental, and because she was married to an Indian she wanted some of her features altered. She also had some breathing problems due to a deviated septum.

Preoperative evaluation On frontal view the nose looked very short and the tip looked blunt, with the eyes being very far apart. On lateral views the nose looked flat and the dorsum was very low. Basal views showed a wide alar base.

The operative goal was to raise the dorsum of the nose, along with a more refined nose tip and a narrower base.

Surgical plan

1. Septoplasty with cartilage harvest
2. Open rhinoplasty with transcolumellar incision
3. Columellar strut with interdomal sutures to narrow tip
4. Dorsal augmentation using an alloplast
5. Alar base reduction.

The preoperative and 3-months postoperative views are given in **Fig. 4**.

Patient 4

This 22-year-old patient wanted to improve the looks of her face. She was concerned that the nose looked very small and also looked retruded relative to the face. She wanted her features to be more defined and the nose to match her face.

Preoperative evaluation On frontal view the nose looked short, the dorsum looked flat, and the eyes were wide apart. The lower third of the nose had

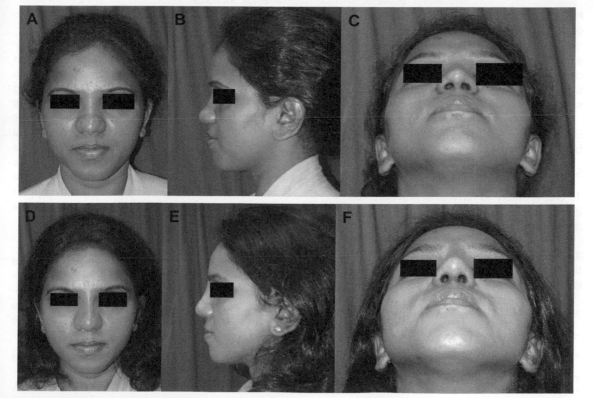

Fig. 3. (A–C) Preoperative views of patient 2. (D–F) The same patient 3 months postoperatively, showing the definition in the nose.

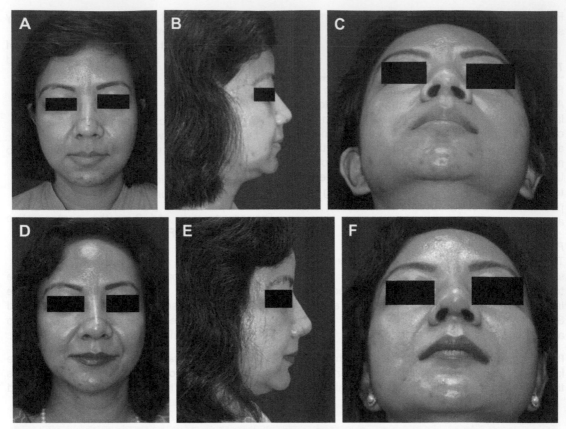

Fig. 4. (*A–C*) Preoperative views of a patient seeking primary rhinoplasty. (*D–F*) The same patient 3 months postoperatively, showing a change in the facial characteristics.

a rhomboid look. On lateral view the dorsum was depressed, the alar base was depressed, and the tip of the nose was upturned. The basal view showed a wide alar base and a short columella.

The operative goal was to achieve a raised longer nose with a defined tip and a raised alar base platform.

Surgical plan

1. Septoplasty to harvest septal cartilage
2. Open rhinoplasty with transcolumellar incision
3. Intraoral upper gingivobuccal incision to place PTFE pyriform rim implants fixed by screws
4. Dorsal augmentation using a silastic implant
5. Septal cartilage for columellar support
6. Shield graft for tip prominence fixed to lower lateral cartilage
7. Wedge resections from the alar base.

Preoperative and 12-month postoperative views are presented in **Fig. 5.**

The Middle Eastern Nose

Middle Eastern and Mediterranean noses usually have specific nasal characteristics. Some of the

noses appear larger than average Caucasian noses. The patients tend to have thick skin with excess fatty tissue, high dorsum with long nose, droopy tip, strong bony and cartilaginous nasal humps, ill-defined and imbalanced nostril tip, acute nasolabial and columellar-labial angles, and wide nasal bones.[21] Many Middle Eastern nose surgery procedures require the surgeon to reduce the height of the dorsum and smooth the nasal humps, along with support of the nasal tip with changes in the cartilaginous framework.

Patient 5

This 37-year-old man consulted the authors because he was concerned about the harsh and boxy look of his nose, which did not complement his face. He was very sure about his requirements, which included downsizing the nose.

Preoperative evaluation The frontal view showed a wide dorsum with thick nasal skin, an overhanging bulbous tip that was slightly deviated, and wide alae. The lateral view showed a hump on the dorsum of the nose along with an

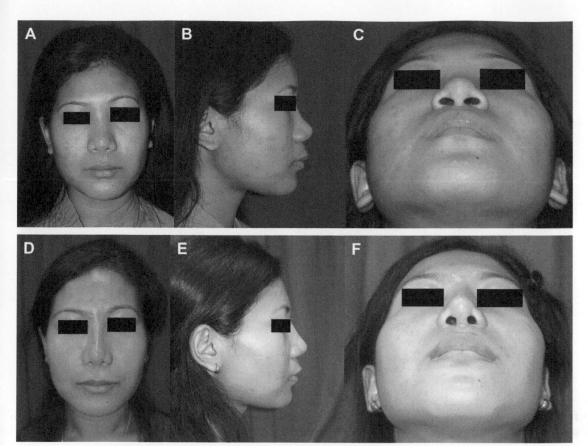

Fig. 5. (*A–C*) Preoperative views of a patient seeking refinement of an Asian nose. (*D–F*) The same patient 1 year postoperatively, showing a well-chiseled nose with a prominent dorsum and a raised nasal platform.

unsupported bulbous nasal tip, almost giving it an overhanging look. The basal view showed a boxy tip with irregular nostril openings.

The operative goal was to narrow the dorsum and make it more straight, raise and support the nasal tip, and reduce the alar openings.

Surgical plan

1. Open rhinoplasty with a transcolumellar incision
2. Septoplasty and harvesting of cartilaginous graft
3. Dorsal hump reduction by rasping
4. Cephalic trim of lower lateral cartilages
5. Columellar strut graft to support the tip and raise it
6. High-low-high transmucosal lateral osteotomy and infracture
7. Interdomal and transdomal sutures
8. Morcelized cartilage graft for the tip
9. Alar base reduction.

Preoperative and 6-month postoperative views are presented in **Fig. 6**.

Patient 6

This 40-year-old married woman presented for improvement of the nose, which was very deviated, wide, and with an overhanging tip. She had Fitzpatrick type 4 skin and did not like her large dorsal hump.

Preoperative evaluation The frontal view showed a prominently deviated dorsum of nose along with a large bulbous nose, and the dorsum appeared wide as well. When the oblique picture was viewed, the true angulation of the dorsum was seen along with a very prominent dorsal hump. There were cartilage prominences on either side of the nasal tip. The basal view showed a very boxy tip, which was also deviated.

The operative goal was to correct the deviation and remove the prominent dorsal hump. The tip also needed to be sharpened.

Surgical plan

1. Septoplasty with harvest of cartilage graft and scoring of the septal cartilage to straighten it
2. Open rhinoplasty with a transcolumellar incision

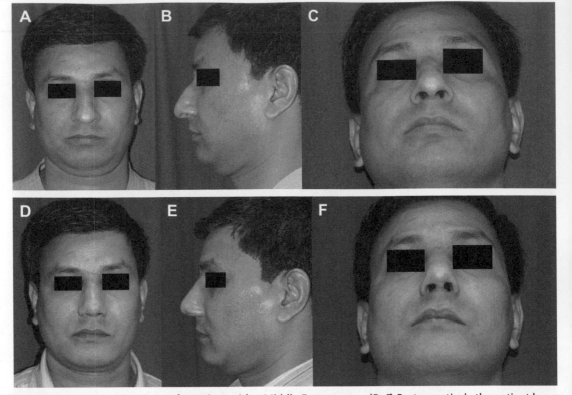

Fig. 6. (*A–C*) Preoperative views of a patient with a Middle Eastern nose. (*D–F*) Postoperatively the patient has an appropriately projecting nose with aesthetically pleasing tip contours.

3. Composite 5-mm dorsal reduction
4. Lateral osteotomy with infracture to straighten the dorsum
5. Open-roof deformity corrected and dorsum straightened with bilateral spreader grafts
6. Cephalic trimming of lower lateral cartilages
7. Columellar strut with interdomal and transdomal sutures
8. Nasal tip further defined by thinning the skin overlying the tip.

Preoperative and 4-month postoperative views are presented in **Fig. 7**.

The Hispanic Nose

Hispanic rhinoplasty procedures cover a wide range of nose types. The Hispanic nose can be a complex amalgamation of various races, as exemplified in the so-called Mestizo nose, which can have characteristics of the Oriental indigenous Indian tribes, African, and/or Spanish white features. At times the nose can be overly protuberant like other Western noses, or other times more akin to the retruded Asian nose, or a combination of both. These noses usually have a thick, sebaceous, soft-tissue envelope, small

osteocartilaginous vault, minimal tip support, a short columellar base, and a broad alar base.[20] Due to a diversity of nasal characteristics, it is essential that a detailed study be performed before proceeding with surgery.

Patient 7

This 35-year-old Hispanic woman request improvement the shape of her nose so that it looked less uneven. She also wanted a reduction in the projection of her nose.

Preoperative evaluation From the frontal view this nose looked perfect except for the bulbous tip, which was overhanging. The lateral view showed the overprojecting tip in a better light, with a normal dorsal height and decreased projection in the radix area and the tip.

The operative goal was to perform a finesse rhinoplasty without lowering the dorsum and achieving sufficient tip projection.

Surgical plan

1. Septoplasty with harvest of cartilage graft
2. Open rhinoplasty with transcolumellar incision
3. Cartilage graft for the radix
4. Cephalic trim of lower lateral cartilage

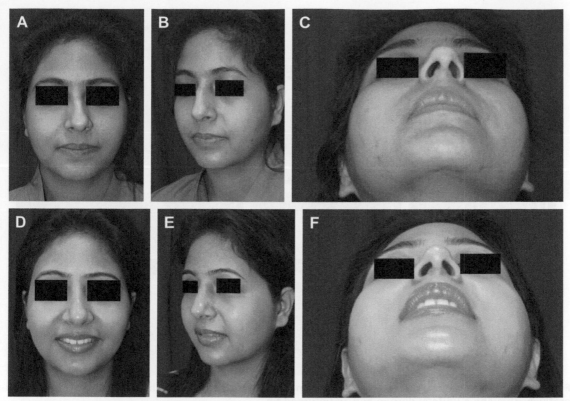

Fig. 7. (*A–C*) Preoperative views of a young woman with a Middle Eastern nose. (*D–F*) The same patient 4 months postoperatively, showing a balanced nose with the dorsum straightened and the nasal tip refined, raised, and projected.

5. Columellar strut used to rotate tip cranially
6. Tip narrowing done using interdomal sutures and defatting the tip skin
7. Alar base wedge resection with internal cinching by sutures.

Preoperative and 1-year postoperative views are shown in **Fig. 8**.

Patient 8

A 28-year-old man wished to improve the shape of his nose. He wanted his nose to be more prominent and narrow. He wanted the tip to be less projecting/droopy and the nasal opening to be more narrow.

Preoperative evaluation The frontal view showed the nose to be wide at the dorsum with a wide alar base, with thick skin. The lateral view showed that the tip was overprojected, with a normal dorsal height. The basal view showed an increased alar width.

The operative goal was to narrow the dorsum and raise it marginally, and to raise and narrow the tip and alar base.

Surgical plan

1. Septoplasty for harvesting of the septal graft
2. Open rhinoplasty with a transcolumellar incision
3. Lateral osteotomy with infracture
4. Dorsal rasping to reduce the dorsal hump palpated
5. Septal cartilage grafts to cover the radix and osteocartilaginous vault
6. Cephalic trim of the lower lateral cartilage
7. Columellar strut support with interdomal sutures
8. Alar base reduction.

Preoperative and 6-month postoperative views are shown in **Fig. 9**.

The Indian Nose

An ill-defined nose is the most commonly encountered problem in clinical practice. These noses typically have a broad lobule and tip, and also lack projection. It is logical to think that the broadness is attributable to lack of projection. In fact in

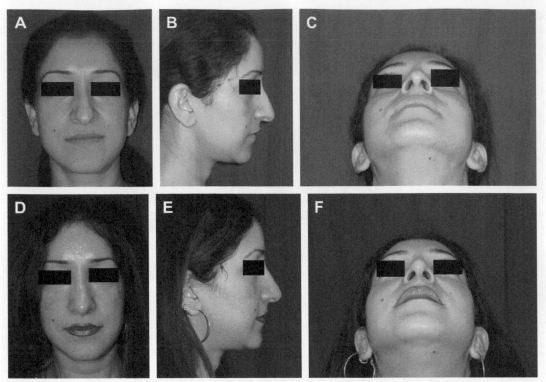

Fig. 8. (*A–C*) Preoperative views of a Hispanic patient with a type 2 nose. (*D–F*) The same patient 1 year postoperatively, showing a uniform dorsum and an upturned tip.

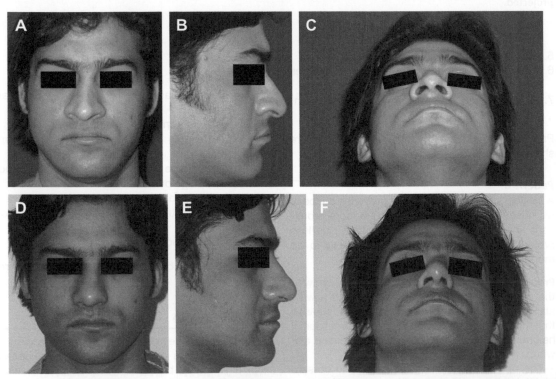

Fig. 9. (*A–C*) Preoperative views of a young Hispanic man. (*D–F*) The same patient 6 months postoperatively, showing a well-balanced nose improved after finesse rhinoplasty.

most cases it is real, and these noses need to be narrowed by osteotomies.

The classic reduction rhinoplasty as described may not be fully applied in the Indian context. The typical Indian nose lacks projection and hence requires augmentation more often than reduction. Some noses may even need reduction at one place and augmentation at the other. Hence cartilage grafting and implants are an integral part of Indian rhinoplasty, and today's surgeon must be

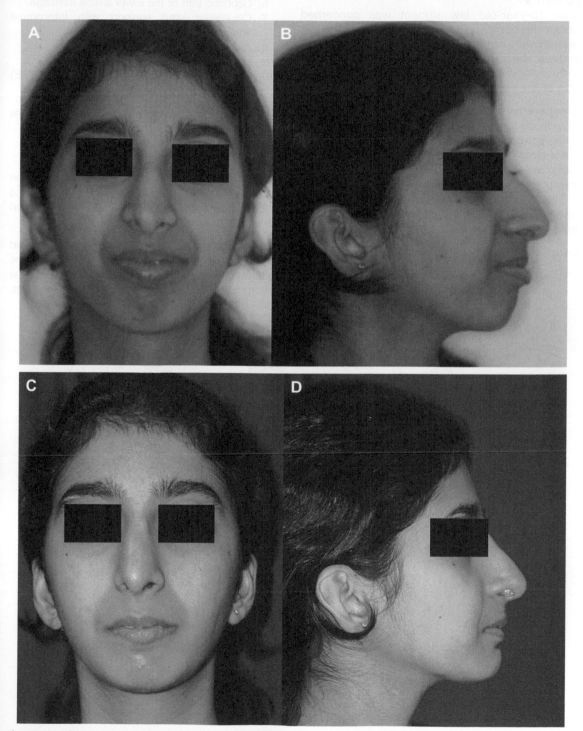

Fig. 10. (*A, B*) Preoperative views of patient 9. (*C, D*) The same patient 6 months postoperatively, showing a good profile.

well versed with the technique and use of cartilage grafts. Usually these patients require associated procedures to improve the facial profile, such as a chin augmentation or changes to the lips.

Patient 9

This 25-year-old law student was concerned about the hump on her nose. Just correcting the hump would not have done much for facial appeal; instead she was advised to consider nasal profile reduction, chin augmentation, and an augmentation of the upper lip.

Preoperative evaluation The frontal view showed a wide dorsum along with an overhanging tip and wide alar base. The lateral view showed the prominent dorsal hump along with a deficiency in the radix area. She had an overprojected nose with thin upper lip and retrogenia.

The operative goal was to downsize the nose and improve the facial profile by improving the lower third of the face.

Surgical plan

1. Septoplasty for harvesting of the cartilage graft

2. Open rhinoplasty with a transcolumellar incision
3. Lateral osteotomy with infracture
4. Dorsal rasping to reduce the dorsal hump
5. Septal cartilage graft to the radix
6. Cephalic trim of the lower lateral cartilage
7. Columellar strut support with interdomal sutures to raise the tip
8. Alar base reduction
9. Lip augmentation using mastoid fascia
10. Chin augmentation using an alloplast (PTFE) done intraorally.

Preoperative and 6-month postoperative views are shown in **Fig. 10**.

Patient 10

This young woman presented for reduction of the nose, as it looked overpowering on her face. She also had a very short chin but was not interested in any augmentation.

Preoperative evaluation The frontal view showed a wide dorsum with a bulbous ill-defined tip. The lateral profile showed the hump on the nose and the overprojection. The basal view showed the boxy tip.

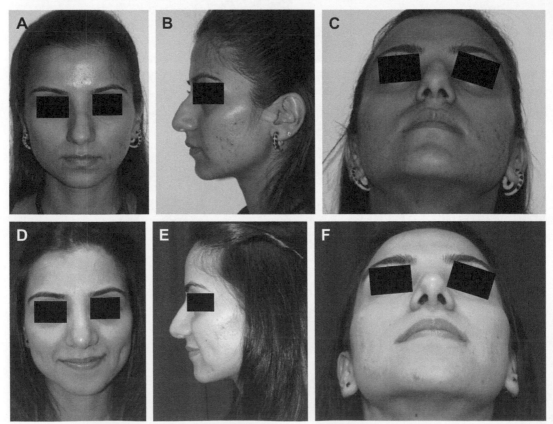

Fig. 11. (A–C) Preoperative views of patient 10. (D–F) The same patient 4 months postoperatively, showing that the areas of concern were fully addressed and improved.

The operative goal was to downsize the nose and to make it more refined in the tip area.

Surgical plan

1. Septoplasty with harvest of cartilage graft
2. Open rhinoplasty with a transcolumellar incision
3. 5-mm dorsal reduction
4. Lateral osteotomy with infracture to narrow the wide dorsal base
5. Open-roof deformity corrected by bilateral spreader grafts
6. Cephalic trimming of lower lateral cartilages
7. Columellar strut with interdomal and transdomal sutures
8. Columellar base narrowed by suturing the foot plates of the lower lateral cartilages.

Preoperative and 4-months postoperative views are presented in **Fig. 11**.

Patient 11
This young patient is being presented to show the extreme form of an Indian nose, for which the

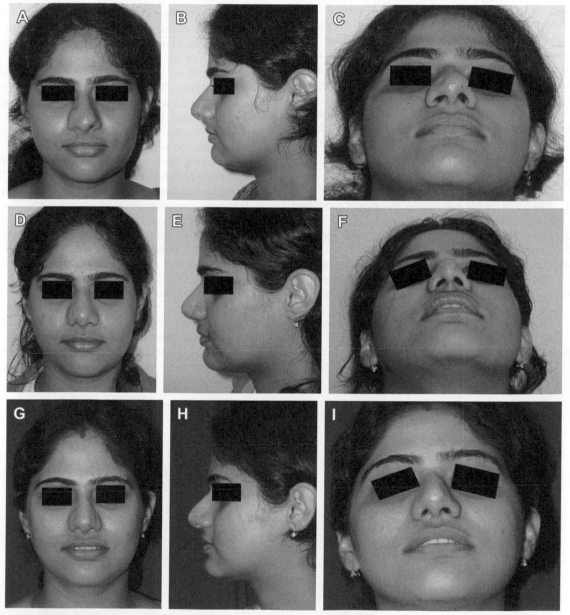

Fig. 12. (*A–C*) Preoperative views of patient 11. (*D–F*) The same patient 6 months postoperatively, showing minimal definition in the tip area because of the thick skin. (*G–I*) The same patient 12 months later, showing significant improvement in the nose definition. The patient is now happy with the results.

surgeon and the patient have to have tremendous patience during the healing phase. This 25-year-old woman presented for improvement of the nose, which looked lopsided. Along with the treatment plan, it was brought to her notice that she had very prominent, thick sebaceous skin of almost rhinophymatous type, which takes a long time to define.

Preoperative evaluation The frontal view showed the nose to be wide at the base of the dorsum, with an ill-defined tip and a wide alar base. The right alar margin was lower than the left. She had thick sebaceous skin. The lateral view shows that the tip projection was adequate, but there was a dorsal hump. The basal view showed an increased alar width with an overhanging and abnormally shaped right lower lateral cartilage. The deviated nasal septum was also seen.

The operative goal was to narrow the dorsum and sharpen it, to raise and narrow the tip, to create a symmetry between the two ala, and to reduce the alar base.

Surgical plan

1. Septoplasty for harvesting the septal graft and correction of the deviation
2. Open rhinoplasty with transcolumellar incision
3. Lateral osteotomy with infracture
4. Dorsal rasping to reduce the dorsal hump
5. Cephalic trim of the lower lateral cartilage
6. Cartilage graft used to support the lateral crura of the right lower lateral cartilage
7. Columellar strut support with interdomal sutures to define and bring the tip up
8. Alar base reduction

9. Fibrofatty soft-tissue reduction and thinning of the skin overlying the tip.

Preoperative views and 6- and 12-month postoperative views are shown in **Fig. 12**.

COMPLICATIONS

The complications seen in rhinoplasty in general are seen in the ethnic population as well. The selective use of implants comes with its own set of problems, such as extrusion (particularly with high-density polyethylene), infection, bony erosion, and displacement (**Fig. 13**).

The authors' preference in select cases is the use of silicone dorsal implants. When used, the pocket size should not be too wide to prevent displacement. In addition, the authors suggest placing 2 holes in the implant, particularly in the part overlying the bony dorsum, to facilitate the creation of the fibrous screw that will anchor the implants. Lastly, the dorsum should be fairly flat, and bony bumps rasped to prevent rocking of the implant, as well making sure whenever possible that the implant rests on a bed of soft tissue/periosteum.

Blistering and hyperpigmentation due to taping of the nose postoperatively is a concern. The suggestion is to keep these patients more closely monitored and remove the tapes if necessary. Bolsters on the nose should be used judiciously, as these patients are very prone to pressure necrosis (**Fig. 14**).

One must carefully evaluate the length and thickness of the nasal bone to avoid bad outcomes when considering osteotomies, as there is such a great variation in the ethnic population. Equally important is the careful evaluation

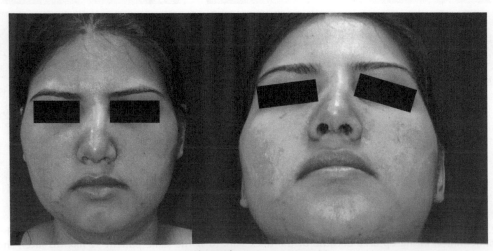

Fig. 13. Displaced silicone dorsal implant at the early postoperative visit.

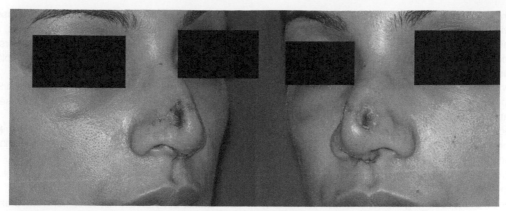

Fig. 14. Full-thickness pressure necrosis from a bolster, secondarily treated by Wolffe graft.

of the height of the septum, particularly when considering septoplasty with or without cartilage harvest, as the septum is usually short in the anteroposterior and cephalocaudal directions. It is extremely important to bear this in mind, so as to keep the L strut at sufficient height in the horizontal component to prevent nasal collapse.

SUMMARY

Rhinoplasty in general is challenging, particularly in the ethnic population. An experienced rhinoplastic surgeon should be able to navigate his or her way through the nuances of the various ethnic subsets. Keeping this in mind and following the established tenets in rhinoplasty, one can expect a pleasing and congruous nose without radically violating ethnicity.

The nasal septum, which forms a very important part of the framework of the nose, is often a culprit contributing to various degrees of asymmetries of the nose with or without the tip being involved. The deviation can exist through its entire course from a cephalad to a caudal direction; however, it is not critical that the very cephalad portion, which may be partly bony, needs to be corrected. The bony spurs that arise from the maxilla should be addressed and trimmed off. Rhinology is well established, and very often patients, particularly those living in the metropolis, suffer from various forms of allergic rhinitis. A preoperative computed tomography scan and an otolaryngology consultation may be necessary to rule out any occult functional problems. The authors believe in a multidisciplinary approach, and in their practice often use the services of an otolaryngologist to help with very difficult septal deviation cases to better serve the patient and spread the risk.

The more difficult and revision rhinoplasties are better done via an open approach, whereas minor tip corrections and/or dorsal humps can be performed by closed rhinoplasty. Due to the thick sebaceous skin cover of most ethnic patients, postoperative swelling of the tip takes a long time to resolve. Furthermore, taping of the tip of the nose at night for several weeks is recommended to reduce edema.

A word of caution is pertinent if dealing with the Middle Eastern, Asian and Indian, and South Asian population with tightly knit families. Patients are often young females accompanied by an entourage of relatives. These patients are very much influenced by the looks of models or actors, and often arrive with their pictures, as these role models drive the cosmetic fashion and trends. It is appropriate to obtain a psychological evaluation for patients whose expectations may be unrealistic or for those requiring multiple surgeries. The authors advise that consultations be very thorough regarding clarity and outcome expectations, to avoid the wrath of the relatives should a patient have a bad outcome. This group of patients places a high priority on confidentiality, and so may not be amenable to preoperative and postoperative photography. The authors advise that under no circumstances should any surgery be undertaken without preoperative and postoperative photos being taken, thus ensuring that the surgeon is adequately insulated against possible litigation. Asian patients, on the other hand, arrive with a limited wish list and rarely pose a problem as a group.

REFERENCES

1. Sheen JH. Aesthetic rhinoplasty. St Louis (MO), Washington, DC, Toronto: The C V Mosby Company; 1987. p. 694–5.
2. Farkas LG, Kolar JC. Anthropometrics and art in the aesthetics of women's faces. Clin Plast Surg 1987; 14:599–616.

3. Fang F, Clapham PJ, Chung KC. A systematic review of interathnic variability in facial dimensions. Plast Reconstr Surg 2011;127:874.

4. American Society of Plastic Surgeons. Briefing paper. Plastic surgery for ethnic patients. Available at: http://www.plasticsurgery.org/Media.html/Media/2011proceduralStatistics/2010Plasticsurgeryproceduralstatistics/2000/2009/2010. National Cosmetic and Reconstructive Plastic Surgery Statistic. Accessed March 5, 2011.

5. Butler PD, Britt LD, Longaker M. Ethnic diversity remains scarce in academic plastic and reconstructive surgery. Plast Reconstr Surg 2009;123:1618–25.

6. Reede JY. A recurring theme: the need for minority physicians. Health Aff (Millwood) 2003;22:91–3.

7. Rappaport NH. Ethnic rhinoplasty. In: Hoefflin SM, editor. New York: Springer – Verlag; 1998. p. 198.

8. Olson S. Mapping human history genes, race and our common origins. New York: Houghton Miffin Company; 2003.

9. Rees TD, Latrenta GS. Aesthetic plastic surgery. Philadelphia: W B Saunders Company; 1994. p. 464, 465.

10. Ofodile FA, James EA. Anatomy of alar cartilages in African-Americans. Plast Reconstr Surg 1997;100:699.

11. Ofodile FA, Bokhari F, Ellis C. The African-American nose. Ann Plast Surg 1993;31:209.

12. Ofodile FA, Bokhari F. The African-American nose. Part II. Ann Plast Surg 1995;34:123.

13. Rohrich RJ, Bolden K. Ethnic rhinoplasty. Clin Plast Surg 2010;37:353–70.

14. Toriumi DM, Pero CD. Asian rhinoplasty. Clin Plast Surg 2010;37:335–52.

15. Ortiz-Monasterio F, Olmedo A. Rhinoplasty on the mestizo nose. Clin Plast Surg 1977;4:89.

16. Ortiz-Monasterio F. Rhinoplasty. Philadelphia: WB Saunders; 1994.

17. Sanchez AE. Rhinoplasty in the "Chata" nose of the Caribbean. Aesthetic Plast Surg 1980;4:196.

18. Milgram LM, Lawson W, Cohen AF. Anthropometric analysis of the female Latino nose. Arch Otolaryngol Head Neck Surg 2003;122:244.

19. Daniel RK. The Hispanic-American nose. In: Rohrich RJ, Gunter JP, Adams WB, editors. Dallas rhinoplasty: nasal surgery by the masters. 2nd edition. St Louis (MO): Quality Medical Publishing; 2007. p. 1197–220.

20. Daniel RK. Hispanic rhinoplasty in the United States, with emphasis on the Mexican-American nose. Plast Reconstr Surg 2003;112:244.

21. Rohrich RJ, Ghavami A. Rhinoplasty for Middle Eastern noses. Plast Reconstr Surg 2009;123:1343.

22. Toriumi DM. New concepts in nasal tip contouring. Arch Facial Plast Surg 2006;8:156.

23. Gunter JP, Rohrich RJ, Friedman RM. Classification and correction of alar-columellar discrepancies in rhinoplasty. Plast Reconstr Surg 1996;97:643.

24. Gunter JP, Friedman RM. Lateral crural strut graft: technique and clinical applications in rhinoplasty. Plast Reconstr Surg 1997;99:943.

25. Rohrich RJ, Raniere J Jr, Ha RY. The alar contour graft: correction and prevention of alar rim deformities in rhinoplasty. Plast Reconstr Surg 2002;109:2495.

26. Ricketts RM. Divine proportion in facial esthetics. Clin Plast Surg 1982;9:401.

27. Guyuron B. The Middle Eastern nose. In: Malory WE Jr, editor. Ethnic consideration for facial aesthetic surgery. Philadelphia: Lippincott-Raven; 1998. p. 363–72.

28. Guyuron B, Ghavami A, Wishnek SM. Components of the short nostril. Plast Reconstr Surg 2005;116:1517.

29. Rohrich RJ, Huynh B, Muzaffar AR, et al. Importance of the depressor septi nasi muscle in rhinoplasty: anatomic study and clinical application. Plast Reconstr Surg 2000;105:376.

30. Poter JP, Olson KL. Analysis of the African American female nose. Plast Reconstr Surg 2003;111:620.

31. Rohrich RJ, Muzaffar AR. Rhinoplasty in the African-American patient. Plast Reconstr Surg 2003;111:1322.

Index

Note: Page numbers of article titles are in **boldface** type.

Oral Maxillofacial Surg Clin N Am 24 (2012) 149–153
doi:10.1016/S1042-3699(12)00009-X
1042-3699/12/$ – see front matter © 2012 Elsevier Inc. All rights reserved.

Moving?

Make sure your subscription moves with you!

To notify us of your new address, find your **Clinics Account Number** (located on your mailing label above your name), and contact customer service at:

Email: journalscustomerservice-usa@elsevier.com

800-654-2452 (subscribers in the U.S. & Canada)
314-447-8871 (subscribers outside of the U.S. & Canada)

Fax number: 314-447-8029

Elsevier Health Sciences Division
Subscription Customer Service
3251 Riverport Lane
Maryland Heights, MO 63043

*To ensure uninterrupted delivery of your subscription, please notify us at least 4 weeks in advance of move.

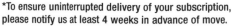

ELSEVIER

Printed and bound by CPI Group (UK) Ltd, Croydon, CR0 4YY

03/10/2024

01040350-0009